Psycho-Oncology in Cancer Survivorship and Health Promotion

PSYCHO-ONCOLOGY CARE SERIES: COMPANION GUIDES
FOR CLINICIANS

Edited by Maggie Watson, PhD, and David Kissane, MD

Published in the Psycho-Oncology Care Series

Management of Clinical Depression and Anxiety

Sexual Health, Fertility, and Relationships in Cancer Care

Psycho- Oncology in Palliative and End of Life Care

Psycho-Oncology in Cancer Survivorship and Health Promotion

Psycho-Oncology in Cancer Survivorship and Health Promotion

Edited by

Maggie Watson, PhD

Visiting Professor, Research Department of Clinical, Health
and Educational Psychology, University College London, UK;
Adjunct Professor of Psychology, Research and Innovation,
University of Southern Queensland, Australia; Editor-in-Chief
Emeritus of Psycho-oncology: Journal of Psychological, Social
and Behavioral Dimensions of Cancer

David Kissane, MD

Professor Emeritus of Palliative Medicine, University of Notre
Dame Australia; Professor Emeritus of Psychiatry, Monash
University, Australia; and Consultation-Liaison Psychiatrist,
Cabrini Health and Monash Health, VIC, Australia

Michael Jefford, PhD

Consultant Medical Oncologist, Director of the Australian
Cancer Survivorship Centre, Peter MacCallum Cancer Centre
in Melbourne, VIC; Professorial Fellow at the University of
Melbourne, VIC, Australia

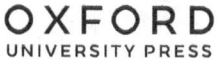
OXFORD
UNIVERSITY PRESS

OXFORD
UNIVERSITY PRESS

Oxford University Press is a department of the University of Oxford.
It furthers the University's objective of excellence in research, scholarship,
and education by publishing worldwide. Oxford is a registered trade mark of
Oxford University Press in the UK and in certain other countries.

Published in the United States of America by Oxford University Press
198 Madison Avenue, New York, NY 10016, United States of America.

CIP data is on file at the Library of Congress.

This material is not intended to be, and should not be considered, a substitute for
medical or other professional advice. Treatment for the conditions described in this
material is highly dependent on the individual circumstances. And, while this material
is designed to offer accurate information with respect to the subject matter covered
and to be current as of the time it was written, research and knowledge about medical
and health issues is constantly evolving and dose schedules for medications are being
revised continually, with new side effects recognized and accounted for regularly.
Readers must therefore always check the product infor-mation and clinical procedures
with the most up-to-date published product information and data sheets provided by
the manufacturers and the most recent codes of conduct and safety regulation. The
publisher and the authors make no representations or warranties to readers, express
or implied, as to the accuracy or completeness of this material. Without limiting the
foregoing, the publisher and the authors make no representations or warranties as to
the accuracy or efficacy of the drug dosages mentioned in the material. The authors
and the publisher do not accept, and expressly disclaim, any responsibility for any
liability, loss, or risk that may be claimed or incurred as a consequence of the use and/
or application of any of the contents of this material.

ISBN 978–0–19–779854–6

DOI: 10.1093/med/9780197798546.001.0001

Printed by Integrated Books International, United States of America

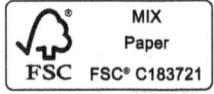

The manufacturer's authorized representative in the EU for product safety is
Oxford University Press España S.A. of Parque Empresarial San Fernando de Henares,
Avenida de Castilla, 2 – 28830 Madrid (www.oup.es/en or product.safety@oup.com).
OUP España S.A. also acts as importer into Spain of products made by the
manufacturer.

Preface

Psycho-oncology is a subspeciality of oncology that focuses on psychosocial problems experienced by cancer patients and their families; it provides evidence-based approaches to management of these specific problems. These *Companion Guides in Psycho-Oncology Care* are intended to make clinical management information accessible to oncology clinical staff, psycho-oncologists, and allied professions seeking to increase their psycho-oncology skills. The material presented here is intended for quick access by clinicians, whatever their discipline, as their patients and families face these challenges, whether medical, psychological, social, or spiritual in nature. This care is directed not only to patients, but also their caregivers and families, to children and adolescents, people from diverse cultural and language backgrounds, the bereaved, and the staff who care for all these people.

The focus here is on those people who now consider themselves cancer survivors. Emotional, social, psychological, and physical support should be available as part of comprehensive cancer care. The aim of this volume is to guide clinicians in providing that support in a skillful way in the survivorship context. The guide is focused on core issues so that the practical manual format can be retained. Topics covered ensure a focus on comprehensive cancer care as it relates to survivorship. This is a pragmatic pocket manual for clinicians who wish to keep up to date with the most recent clinical literature across the psycho-oncology spectrum and is the fourth in the successful International Psycho-Oncology Society series of Companion Guides for Clinicians.

Because this volume focuses primarily on survivorship issues, a wide range of symptoms and unmet needs, as well as broader issues, will be discussed, including

- Psychological issues, including anxiety and adjustment disorder, fear of cancer recurrence or progression, and depressive disorder
- Cognitive impairment
- Practical issues, particularly return to work or study, and financial issues
- The spiritual and cultural context of care
- Focus on survivors of cancer in childhood, during adolescence, and in young adults
- Rehabilitation, health promotion, and self-management.

The authors of this *Companion Guide* are clinicians and researchers with many years of experience in the care of patients with cancer and their families. We thank them for sharing this expertise. As editors, we also thank the staff of Oxford University Press for their support and the International Psycho-Oncology Society for assistance with distribution of these official society clinical guides.

The psychosocial care of cancer patients and their families is a basic human right. We hope that the readers of this volume will find it helpful to advance the quality of this care delivery to enrich the lives of all patients with cancer and their families.

Maggie Watson, PhD
David Kissane, MD
Michael Jefford, PhD

Contents

Contributors

Tim Ahles, PhD
Department of Psychiatry and
   Behavioral Sciences, Memorial
   Sloan Kettering Cancer Center,
   New York, NY, USA

Tatsuo Akechi, MD, PhD
Department of Psychiatry and
   Cognitive-Behavioral Medicine,
   Graduate School of Medical
   Sciences, Nagoya City University,
   Nagoya, Japan

Susanne Oksbjerg Dalton, PhD
Danish Cancer Institute, Cancer
   Survivorship, Copenhagen,
   Denmark; Danish Research
   Center for Equality in Cancer
   (COMPAS), Department for
   Clinical Oncology & Palliative
   Care, Zealand University
   Hospital, Næstved, Denmark

Anne-Sophie Darlington, PhD
School of Health Sciences,
   University of Southampton,
   Southampton, United Kingdom

Jayita Deodhar, MD
Department of Palliative Medicine,
   Tata Memorial Hospital, Mumbai,
   India; Homi Bhabha National
   Institute, Mumbai, India

Saskia F. A. Duijts, PhD
Department of Research &
   Development, Netherlands
   Comprehensive Cancer
   Organisation (IKNL), Utrecht;
   Department of Medical
   Psychology, Amsterdam University
   Medical Centre; Cancer Center
   Amsterdam, Cancer Treatment
   and Quality of Life, Amsterdam,
   The Netherlands

Joanne Fardell, PhD
Behavioural Sciences Unit, School
   of Clinical Medicine, University
   of New South Wales Medicine &
   Health, UNSW Sydney; Western
   Sydney Youth Cancer Service,
   Westmead Hospital, New South
   Wales, Australia

Margaret I. Fitch, PhD
Bloomberg Faculty of Nursing,
   University of Toronto,
   Toronto, Canada

Claire Foster, PhD
Centre for Psychosocial
   Research in Cancer, University
   of Southampton, United
   Kingdom

Daisuke Fujisawa, MD, PhD
National Cancer Center, Institute
   for Cancer Control, Chuo-ku,
   Tokyo, Japan

Mu-Hsing Ho, PhD
School of Nursing, Li Ka
   Shing Faculty of Medicine,
   University of Hong Kong, Hong
   Kong, China

Doris Howell, PhD
Princess Margaret Cancer Research
   Institute, Toronto, Canada

Michael Jefford, PhD
Australian Cancer Survivorship
   Centre, Centre for Health
   Services Research, and
   Department of Medical
   Oncology, Peter MacCallum
   Cancer Centre, Melbourne,
   Victoria, Australia

Christoffer Johansen, MD, PhD
CASTLE, Cancer Late Effects
 Research Unit, Oncology,
 Rigshospitalet,
University of Copenhagen,
 Copenhagen, Denmark

Youngmee Kim, PhD
Department of Psychology,
 University of Miami, Coral
 Gables, FL, USA

Alex King, DClinPsy
Department of Surgery and Cancer,
 Imperial College, London,
 United Kingdom

David Kissane, AC, MD
School of Medicine, University of
 Notre Dame Australia, Sydney,
 NSW; Department of Psychiatry,
 Monash University, VIC; and
 Psycho-oncology Service, Cabrini
 Health and Monash Health, VIC,
 Australia

Bogda Koczwara, PhD
Australian Research Centre for
 Cancer Survivorship, Faculty of
 Medicine and Health, Health
 Translation Hub, University of
 New South Wales, Sydney, NSW,
 Australia

Wendy Lam, PhD
Division of Behavioral Sciences,
 School of Public Health, LKS
 Faculty of Medicine, University
 of Hong Kong, Hong Kong
 SAR, China

Sophie Lebel, PhD
School of Psychology, University
 of Ottawa, Ottawa,
 Ontario, Canada

Anne Maas, PhD
Princess Máxima Center for
 Pediatric Oncology, Utrecht, The
 Netherlands

Daniel McFarland, DO
Department of Psychiatry, University
 of Rochester Medical Center,
 Rochester, NY, USA;
Wilmot Cancer Center, Rochester,
 NY, USA

Anja Mehnert-Theuerkauf, PhD
Department of Medical Psychology
 and Medical Sociology, University
 Medical Center Leipzig, Leipzig,
 Germany

Gozde Ozakinci, PhD
Division of Psychology, Faculty of
 Natural Sciences, University of
 Stirling, Stirling, Scotland, United
 Kingdom

Patricia A. Parker, PhD
Department of Psychiatry &
 Behavioral Sciences, Memorial
 Sloan Kettering Cancer Center,
 New York, NY, USA

Julia H. Rowland, PhD
Smith Center for Healing & the Arts,
 Washington, DC, USA

Ben Smith PhD
The Daffodil Centre, The University
 of Sydney, A Joint Venture with
 Cancer Council NSW, Sydney,
 NSW, Australia

Kelly R. Tan, PhD
Department of Health and
 Community Systems, University
 of Pittsburgh School of Nursing,
 Pittsburgh, PA, USA

Janette Vardy, PhD
Concord Clinical School, Faculty of
 Medicine and Health, University
 of Sydney, NSW; Sydney Cancer
 Survivorship Centre, Concord
 Repatriation General Hospital,
 Sydney, NSW, Australia

Claire E. Wakefield, PhD
School of Clinical Medicine, Faculty
of Medicine, UNSW Sydney,
NSW, Australia;
Division of Quality of Life and
Pediatric Palliative Care,
Department of Pediatrics,
Stanford Medicine Children's
Health, Palo Alto, CA, USA

Maggie Watson, PhD
Research Department of Clinical,
Education and Health Psychology,
University College London,
UK; Research and Innovation,
University of Southern
Queensland, Queensland,
Australia

Lori Wiener, PhD
Pediatric Oncology Branch, Center
for Cancer Research, National
Cancer Institute, National
Institutes of Health, Bethesda,
MD, USA

Chapter 1

Managing Long-Term and Late Effects in the Survivorship Context

Issues and Overview of Psychosocial Care

Michael Jefford, David Kissane, and Maggie Watson

Learning Objectives

After reading this chapter, the clinician will be able to:

1. Understand terminology, prevalence, and the breadth of issues experienced by cancer survivors.
2. Recognize evidence-based core components for psychosocial survivorship care.
3. Implement key investigations and assessment methods.
4. Understand the potential value of survivorship care plans (SCPs).
5. Recognize evidence to support different models of survivorship care.
6. Implement professional multidisciplinary processes needed to deliver quality comprehensive survivorship care.

Background Evidence

Following the introduction of chemotherapy in the 1950s, many previously fatal cancers became treatable and some curable, particularly cancers diagnosed in childhood. Follow-up studies, however, showed that many survivors experience very significant adverse consequences due to cancer treatments. This marked the beginning of significant focus on the post-treatment survivorship phase. The US National Coalition for Cancer Survivorship, formed in 1986, provided the broad, inclusive definition of "cancer survivor." Other key milestones were the formation of the Office of Cancer Survivorship within the US National Cancer Institute (NCI) in 1996; the launch of the US Institute of Medicine (IOM) report "From Cancer Patient to Cancer Survivor, Lost in

Transition," in 2006; the development of the *Journal of Cancer Survivorship* in 2007; and England's National Cancer Survivorship Initiative in 2010. This led to the development of policies for structured survivorship care to support patients over the longer term in relation to their cancer experience and treatment late effects. Health promotion is also a key component of optimal survivorship care, with studies showing improvements in health risk factors and long-term outcomes. SCPs remain a recommended component of comprehensive care.

Definition of Survivor

The US NCI notes, "an individual is considered a cancer survivor from the time of diagnosis through the balance of life. There are many types of survivors, including those living with cancer and those free of cancer. This concept is meant to capture a population of those with a history of cancer rather than to provide a label that may or may not resonate with individuals."[1] The term "survivor" is rejected by some patient and consumer groups who prefer alternatives such as "living with and beyond cancer" or "life after cancer." The term "survivor" may not translate as broadly in languages other than English.[2] The NCI also notes[1] "There is no one face or kind of cancer survivor. Some have been treated for their cancer and remain cancer-free, while others continue to live with cancer. The experiences and goals of care for each cancer survivor are unique and dynamic."

Particularly as a result of novel treatments, including immunotherapies and targeted treatments, there are growing numbers of people with "treatable but not curable" cancers.[3] However, for the purpose of survivorship care development plans, it is helpful to retain the broad generic definition provided by the NCI.

Prevalence

As a result of the growing and aging population, improved cancer detection, and more effective treatments, the number of cancer survivors is growing substantially. Most are long-term survivors. The number of American cancer survivors has risen from 3 million in 1971 to an estimated 18.6 million in 2025.[4] The most prevalent survivor groups are those with a personal history of breast cancer, prostate cancer, melanoma, colorectal cancer, and thyroid cancer. Most (70%) have survived at least 5 years post initial diagnosis; 49% more than 10 years, 22% more than 20, and 11% of US survivors have survived 25 years or more post diagnosis. There are similar large numbers of survivors in Europe, with an estimated 23.7 million survivors in 2020, representing 5% of the total population.[5]

As noted above, some survivors may be living with advanced or metastatic cancer, and a substantial proportion of these will have "treatable but not curable" cancers. The number of survivors in this category cannot be accurately quantified but has been estimated to be more than 600,000 in the United States and between 100,000 and 200,000 in England.[3] These survivors may live for many years with cancer and may have periods on and off treatment. For decades, this grouping has included a sizeable number with metastatic breast, prostate, and hematological cancers, such as low-grade lymphoma.

With more recent treatments many with advanced cancer who previously had a poor prognosis (e.g., those with metastatic melanoma and metastatic lung cancers) are now surviving many years, some of whom may even be cured.

Another important group to note are survivors of cancer experienced in childhood or as an adolescent or young adult.[6] Although cancer in these age groups is uncommon, these groups experience the greatest risk for ongoing (long-term) and delayed-onset (late) effects and may be in a post-treatment survivorship phase for many decades (see also Chapter 9).

A large number of people with an inherited genetic risk are at high risk of developing cancer and share many issues with cancer survivors, including worry about cancer development, the need to make complex risk reduction decisions, concern for those close to them, and a focus on remaining well. They may also have practical concerns, such as difficulty obtaining life and health insurance.

Notably, the above estimates do not include the millions of informal caregivers who provide unpaid support to cancer survivors. Caregivers experience substantial burdens and may have unmet needs for psychological support and financial assistance, and for training on how to support their loved ones[6] (see also Chapter 6).

Presenting Problems

Issues for Cancer Survivors

Survivors of different types and stages of cancer report varied survivorship issues.[7-9] They commonly report both symptoms and unmet needs during the treatment period and in the post-treatment phase.[8] Domains of unmet needs can include activities of daily living, communication, economic, information, physical, psychological, psychosocial, supportive care, sexuality, spirituality, and transportation.[8] A greater number of people in the post-treatment phase appear to report unmet needs compared to other phases of the cancer continuum.[8]

From studies that used the Supportive Care Needs Survey, commonly reported unmet needs include[8]

- **Psychological domain:** Fears about the cancer spreading, concerns about the worries of those closest, and uncertainty about the future.
- **Information domain:** Being informed about things you can do to help yourself get well, being adequately informed about benefits and side effects of treatment, and information about remission status.
- **Physical and daily living domain:** Pain, not being able to do things you used to do, and work around the home.

For people affected by metastatic cancer, both survivors and caregivers may experience substantial unmet needs.[10] Childhood and adolescent survivors, even when cured of their initial cancer, carry a substantially increased risk of chronic health conditions and premature death.[6] A study of 5,522 survivors of childhood cancer who underwent comprehensive follow-up found the cumulative incidence of a severe, disabling, life-threatening, or fatal chronic condition was 96%.[11] By age 50, survivors had, on average, 17.1 chronic health conditions, including 4.7 graded as severe, disabling, life-threatening, or fatal.[11] The cumulative burden in these survivors was nearly double that of community controls. Common late effects include cardiovascular disease, respiratory problems, endocrine abnormalities, and second cancers[6] (see also Chapter 9).

Current Care and Follow-Up Issues

Guidelines recommend that survivors receive some form of follow-up care after completing treatment for cancer.[7] The traditional specialist-led model of care continues to be the most prevalent and tends to be medically focused (oncologist- or hematologist-led), delivered in a specialist cancer setting or in a hospital, and often following survivors for around 5 years post treatment.[9,12] This model tends to focus on surveillance for possible cancer recurrence and physical symptoms, with less attention paid to screening for and responding to psychosocial issues, health promotion, management of comorbid illness, and effective care coordination.[12,13]

A recent survey by the International Psycho-Oncology Society focused on psychosocial care for cancer survivors across the world.[14] Thirty-seven countries were represented, with 40% of responses from low- and middle-income countries. Participants reported that the most common elements of survivorship care related to prevention and management of recurrent or new cancers (74%), physical long-term or late effects (59%), and chronic medical conditions (53%), whereas surveillance and management of psychosocial late effects (27%) and psychosocial and supportive care (25%) were least common. Barriers to more holistic, comprehensive care included a predominant focus on medical treatment rather than on broader post-treatment survivorship care and a lack of allied health providers to deliver psychosocial care. Enablers included having policy and guidance documents focusing on psychosocial care for survivors.[14]

A key US report from the IOM brought major focus on the issues experienced by cancer survivors, particularly in the post-treatment survivorship phase, and catalyzed an international surge in research and practice change toward better survivorship care.[9] The IOM report defined four essential components of survivorship care:

1. Prevention of recurrent and new cancers and of other late effects,
2. Surveillance not just for cancer spread, recurrence, or second cancers, but also for medical and psychosocial long-term and late effects,
3. Interventions to deal with the consequences of cancer and its treatment, including medical problems such as lymphedema; symptoms, such as pain and fatigue; distress experienced by both survivors and caregivers; and concerns related to employment, insurance, and disability,
4. Coordination between all healthcare providers to ensure that survivors' health needs are met. The IOM report also made 10 recommendations (see Box 1.1).

Box 1.1 IOM Report: Ten Recommendations for Survivorship Care

1	Raising awareness of the needs of survivors, establishing survivorship as a distinct phase, and acting to deliver appropriate care for survivors
2	Providing survivors with a treatment summary and a survivorship care plan detailing plans for follow-up
3	Developing and utilizing evidence-based guidelines, assessment tools, and screening instruments to identify and manage effects of cancer and treatment
4	Developing and implementing measures of quality survivorship care
5	Testing models of coordinated interdisciplinary care
6	Ensuring that comprehensive cancer plans include focus on survivorship care
7	Expanding education for health professionals to better care for survivors
8	Eliminating discrimination and minimizing adverse effects of cancer on work participation and supporting survivors to return to work
9	Ensuring that survivors have access to the healthcare they need, including necessary health insurance
10	Increasing support for survivorship research

Source: National Research Council. *From Cancer Patient to Cancer Survivor: Lost in Transition*. National Academies Press; 2006. https://doi.org/10.17226/11468.

Significant progress has been made since the 2006 IOM report; however, these recommendations are still highly relevant internationally.

Models of Care

The IOM suggested that various organizations "should support demonstration programs to test models of coordinated, interdisciplinary survivorship care in diverse communities and across systems of care."[9] The report noted that "several promising models for delivering survivorship care are emerging, including:

- a shared-care model in which specialists work collaboratively with primary care providers
- a nurse-led model in which nurses take responsibility for cancer-related follow-up care with oversight from physicians
- specialized survivorship clinics in which multidisciplinary care is offered at one site."[9]

Recent reviews examined the effectiveness of shared care and care that is led by primary care providers and nurses.[12,13] Most studies have been conducted in Western, developed countries and involved survivors of breast, gynecological, colorectal, prostate, lung, and esophageal cancers. Many studies were designed to show that novel models produce similar outcomes to traditional, specialist-led care. Generally, the focus of the intervention has been on adherence to recommended surveillance testing without significant focus on the breadth of survivorship care. Study endpoints focused on adherence to testing and observation of cancer recurrences although also measured, to an extent, physical symptoms, psychosocial effects, satisfaction and quality of life, and costs.[12,13] Together, alternate models of care seem as effective as traditional, specialist-led care according to the endpoints assessed. These models may also be cheaper for the healthcare system and for patients themselves.[12,13]

Multidisciplinary survivorship clinics have also been developed. These may be a one-off consultative service or offer longitudinal care. The latter has been utilized to support people at risk of late effects. Such services may include a range of medical specialists (pediatric and adult oncologist and hematologists, cardiology, endocrinology, etc.), cancer nurses, psychologists and psychiatrists, and a range of allied health providers (including social workers, speech pathologists, occupational therapists, and exercise physiologists). Advantages include survivors' needs being comprehensively assessed and managed and a major focus sustained on surveillance and late effects. Disadvantages include increased resource requirements, limited capacity/availability, and separation of survivorship care from routine care. There are limited data regarding the evaluation of this model.

England provides the best example of a widespread shift in the model of care.[12,15] Here, particularly for highly prevalent cancers (breast, prostate, and colorectal), there has been a shift to "personalized stratified follow-up" in which a proportion of patients do not have regular oncology follow-up appointments but are supported to self-manage and have remote monitoring that adheres to recommended surveillance testing.

Survivors also receive "personalized care and support planning" comprising holistic needs assessments, an end-of-treatment summary, health and well-being information and support, and a cancer care review in the primary care setting.

For patients thought not appropriate for self-management with remote monitoring, a shared care model might be used. A few survivors might be better managed through a hospital-based multidisciplinary team.[12,15] Publicly reported data suggest that, in the United Kingdom, the majority of hospital Trusts already have pathways to support personalized care and planning and stratified follow-up.[12] The focus on health and well-being represents a deliberate and systematic approach to incorporate health promoting activities (see also Chapter 11).

Investigations for Key Differential Diagnosis

The IOM report recommended that "health care providers should use systematically developed evidence-based clinical practice guidelines, assessment tools, and screening instruments to help identify and manage late effects of cancer and its treatment."[9]

As described in subsequent chapters, a number of tools have been developed to screen and assess for psychosocial concerns. It is also important to consider how to implement a whole pathway to routinely identify and manage survivors' issues.[16] The pathway should consider how patients complete a screening tool, the process for further assessment, referral to services for management, and ongoing rescreening.[16] Ideally, organizations should include outcome measurements that might assess survivors' quality of life and functional rehabilitation.

Emery and colleagues provide a guide for a general survivorship-focused consultation.[7] Elements include reviewing details of the cancer history, considering risk of recurrence and reviewing local guidelines for surveillance, asking about common problems, discussing lifestyle factors, and addressing and managing chronic medical conditions.

The US National Comprehensive Cancer Network (NCCN) has developed a survivorship guideline that includes a 29-question survivorship assessment focusing on cardiac health, anxiety, depression, trauma and distress, cognitive function, fatigue, lymphoedema, pain, hormone-related symptoms, sexual health, fertility, sleep disorders, healthy lifestyle, immunizations and infections, and employment/return to work.[17] The checklist (see Box 1.2) has face validity and has been widely used, although not further validated.

Survivorship Care Plans

Based on the IOM report,[9] the SCP ideally should include

- A summary of the person's cancer diagnosis and treatments,
- Information about current symptoms, issues, and concerns,
- Suggested follow-up schedule,

Box 1.2 Survivorship Assessment Recommended by the NCCN

Referenced with permission from the NCCN Clinical Practice Guidelines in Oncology (NCCN Guidelines®) for Survivorship V.2.2024. © National Comprehensive Cancer Network, Inc. 2024. All rights reserved. Accessed January 2025. To view the most recent and complete version of the guideline, go online to NCCN.org. NCCN makes no warranties of any kind whatsoever regarding their content, use or application and disclaims any responsibility for their application or use in any way.

- Information about symptoms to be alert for and about possible late effects,
- Approaches to remain well, including screening and health promotion, recommendations, and
- Information about support services.

Although survivors and many providers value care plans, there is limited evidence to support their impact on clinical outcomes. Several randomized controlled trials have been conducted about the use of SCPs.[18,19] but there have not been consistent benefits found across a number of health and healthcare delivery outcomes. Importantly, no harm has occurred. They may improve survivors' adherence to medical recommendations and healthcare professionals' knowledge of survivorship care and late effects.[18] Reviews note major heterogeneity in terms of the content of SCPs, how they are used in practice, and study endpoints. They have provided useful recommendations regarding how to improve research studies examining the impact of SCPs.[18,19]

🔍 Key Point

The Survivorship Care Plan (SCP) should be given to the survivor themselves and shared with other members of the care team, including the person's primary care provider. Ideally, the care plan is based on a needs assessment and patient priorities, discussed in a dedicated clinical consultation, and regularly updated. Receipt of SCPs has been included in quality standards. Whatever the institutional model of survivorship care, an end-of-treatment consultation marks a transition to survivorship care and supports continuity of care.[20]

Measuring Outcomes

The IOM report recommended that "quality of survivorship care measures should be developed . . . and quality assurance programs implemented by health systems to monitor and improve the care that all survivors receive."[9] Nekhlyudov and colleagues developed a "Quality of cancer survivorship care framework."[20] "Surveillance and management of psychosocial effects" is included as one of five core aspects of healthcare delivery. Subdomains include psychological, financial/employment, and interpersonal. A separate domain focuses on health promotion, which considers disease prevention, cancer screening, smoking cessation, weight management, diet and physical activity, and other lifestyle behaviors. Suggested outcome measures include health-related quality of life, function, healthcare utilization, costs, and survival.[20] Recently (2024), national cancer survivorship standards have been developed in the United States[21] based on a quality framework developed in Australia.[22]

The standards are arranged in three domains of health system policy, process, and evaluation/assessment.

1. Examples within the policy domain include that the organization should have a policy that specifies "establishment or existence of a survivorship program either on-site, through telehealth, or by referral" and "an outline for the provision of information for support services (e.g., navigators, social work, interpreters) for survivors based on their needs (including but not limited to health, insurance, financial literacy,

and disability status), including survivors from diverse and underserved backgrounds."[21]

2. Examples in the process domain are that survivors be "assessed at multiple points in their follow-up care for emotional and psychological effects of cancer and its treatment and provided with treatment and/or referrals"[21] and "assessed for practical and social effects of cancer and its treatment (e.g., social risks, health-related social needs, education and employment/return to work or school) and provided with resources and/or referrals"[21] as well as "assessed for lifestyle behaviours and provided with recommended strategies for management and appropriate referrals or education as needed (e.g., smoking cessation, diet/nutrition counselling, promoting physical activity)."[21]

3. With respect to evaluation and assessment, the standards note that an organization should have a process to collect data on "survivors' patient-reported outcomes, including quality of life, and experiences of survivorship care" also "survivors' functional capacity" and "survivors' return to previous participation in paid and unpaid work/school/productive activities of living."[21]

Clinical Management

Survivorship care begins from diagnosis. Many issues that impact life after cancer need to be considered early and proactively, for example:

- Symptom and needs assessment
- Early screening, assessment, and management of psychosocial issues to help prevent or reduce these in the post-treatment period
- Consideration of—and ideally prevention of—long-term and late effects, such as infertility
- Consideration of services available in the cancer setting and/or in the community, to meet identified needs
- Discussion of the expected model of follow-up throughout the treatment phase
- Periodic assessment of information needs; toward the end of treatment, survivors can be provided with general and more specific information (relevant to type of cancer or individual treatments)
- Consideration of how to support self-management, with a focus on health promotion
- Clarification of the role of different providers and provision of a tool for care coordination.

Case Study

A 46-year-old woman with a screen-detected early breast cancer was treated with wide local excision and adjuvant radiation. She has recently started hormonal therapy, with a plan to continue this for 10 years. She works at a library and is a single parent, with an adult daughter. The hospital social worker helped her with financial advice and worked with her and her employer on a return to work plan. She has been troubled by hot flashes and reports worries about the cancer coming back, concerns for the future, and worry about her daughter also getting breast cancer. Her follow-up is shared between a nurse practitioner at the hospital and her general practitioner (GP), both of whom alternate visits. She was provided with an SCP by her nurse practitioner, which included information on potential late effects from cancer treatments. This has also been shared with her GP. They have a shared electronic record. The patient is in touch with a breast cancer charity and has support from a peer volunteer. The nurse practitioner has been helping her with the adjuvant hormonal therapy, including how to manage hot flashes. They discussed psychological issues, including that these are common in cancer survivors. A psychologist from the GP practice now works with the patient and this will be reviewed by the GP.

Professional Issues and Service Implementation

Recording and Communicating

An SCP may be useful for survivors, caregivers, and health professionals. Clinicians and health providers should also consider the following:

1. Patients should be asked about their information preferences, which should be documented and followed by clinicians and health providers.
2. Non-governmental organizations and cancer charities often have excellent general survivorship information.
3. SCPs should provide specific information relevant to the individual survivor.
4. The SCP should also clarify clinician and health provider roles and responsibilities.
5. Use of screening tools and question prompt lists (see Further Reading section) can help survivors to identify issues and supports patient-centered care.
6. As in other settings, audio recordings of consultations may promote greater recall.[23]

Ensure that all relevant clinicians and services are informed of the SCP to ensure coordinated care across hospital and community services.

Legal Responsibilities

Patients have a right to be informed about serious effects of treatment, which might include the risk of developing another cancer as a consequence of cancer treatments, cardiac and lung damage, fertility, sexual and endocrine dysfunction, and long-term consequences (some of which are currently poorly understood) from immunotherapy and other newer treatments.

Cultural Issues

The term "cancer survivor" does not translate to a similar term in many languages. Other terms may be needed to describe individuals and the post-treatment phase. Cancer carries stigma in many cultures. People, even those cancer-free, may be shunned from previous social situations. There may be cultural differences when discussing finances, relationships, and sexuality. Providers should seek out culturally appropriate information and support services. When patients belong to culturally and linguistically diverse communities, the use of a professional interpreter is critical to optimizing understanding. This applies to the translation of an SCP into the first language of the index patient.

Common Ethical Dilemmas

Survivors have disparate outcomes and experiences based on factors such as socioeconomic position, income, geography, and race. Inequitable access and disparate outcomes may also arise due to variable insurance coverage.

Clinicians express concern about the extent to which they should discuss late effects that may have a low risk of occurrence, knowing that full disclosure of the range of possible late effects can potentially burden a patient. Clinicians can ask the patient how much detail they like to receive and provide written information that allows the patient the option of reading this if they wish to do so.

Policies for Clinical Services

It is important to develop policies for survivorship care because they act as a platform and can define quality survivorship care. Increasingly, standards are being developed to define quality survivorship care. Accreditation standards for hospitals and cancer centers will predictably require a survivorship program as a necessary component of their care.

Teams and Supervision

Teams will comprise a mix of medical, nursing, and allied health disciplines, requiring significant administrative support and appropriate training and supervision. Supervision may come from a relevant senior specialist from the appropriate discipline and provide support to staff in both acute and primary care settings.

References

1. https://cancercontrol.cancer.gov/ocs/definitions. Accessed Feb 1 2025.

2. O'Callaghan C, Schofield P, Butow P, et al. "I might not have cancer if you didn't mention it": A qualitative study on information needed by culturally diverse cancer survivors. Support Care Cancer. 2016;24:409–418

3. Lai-Kwon J, Heynemann S, Hart NH, et al. Evolving landscape of metastatic cancer survivorship: Reconsidering clinical care, policy, and research priorities for the modern era. J Clin Oncol. 2023;41:3304–3310.

4. Wagle NS, Nogueira L, Devasia TP, et al. Cancer treatment and survivorship statistics, 2025. CA Cancer J Clin. 2025 Jul-Aug;75(4):308–340. doi: 10.3322/caac.70011. Epub 2025 May 30.

5. De Angelis R, Demuru E, Baili P, et al. Complete cancer prevalence in Europe in 2020 by disease duration and country (EUROCARE-6): A population-based study. Lancet Oncol. 2024;25:293–307.

6. Tonorezos ES, Cohn RJ, Glaser AW, et al. Long-term care for people treated for cancer during childhood and adolescence. Lancet. 2022;399:1561–1572.

7. Emery J, Butow P, Lai-Kwon J, et al. Management of common clinical problems experienced by survivors of cancer. Lancet. 2022;399:1537–1550.

8. Harrison JD, Young JM, Price MA, et al. What are the unmet supportive care needs of people with cancer? A systematic review. Support Care Cancer. 2009;17:1117–1128.

9. National Research Council. *From Cancer Patient to Cancer Survivor: Lost in Transition.* National Academies Press; 2006. https://doi.org/10.17226/11468.

10. Hart NH, Crawford-Williams F, Crichton M, et al. Unmet supportive care needs of people with advanced cancer and their caregivers: A systematic scoping review. Crit Rev Oncol Hematol. 2022;176:103728.

11. Bhakta N, Liu Q, Ness KK, et al. The cumulative burden of surviving childhood cancer: An initial report from the St Jude Lifetime Cohort Study (SJLIFE). Lancet. 2017;390:2569–2582.

12. Jefford M, Howell D, Li Q, et al. Improved models of care for cancer survivors. Lancet. 2022;399:1551–1560.

13. Chan RJ, Crawford-Williams F, Crichton M, et al. Effectiveness and implementation of models of cancer survivorship care: An overview of systematic reviews. J Cancer Surviv. 2023;17:197–221.

14. Signorelli C, Hoeg BL, Asuzu C, et al. International survey of psychosocial care for cancer survivors in low-/middle- and high-income countries: Current practices, barriers, and facilitators to care. JCO Glob Oncol. 2024;10:e2300418.

15. Jefford M, Rowland J, Grunfeld E, et al. Implementing improved post-treatment care for cancer survivors in England, with reflections from Australia, Canada and the USA. Br J Cancer. 2013;108:14–20.

16. Stout NL, Alfano CM, Liu R, et al. Implementing a clinical pathway for needs assessment and supportive care interventions. JCO Oncol Pract. 2024;20:1173–1181.

17. NCCN Guidelines Version 1.2024 Survivorship. https://www.nccn.org/guidelines/guidelines-detail?category=3&id=1466

18. Hill RE, Wakefield CE, Cohn RJ, et al. Survivorship care plans in cancer: A meta-analysis and systematic review of care plan outcomes. Oncologist. 2020;25:e351–e372.

19. Jacobsen PB, DeRosa AP, Henderson TO, et al. Systematic review of the impact of cancer survivorship care plans on health outcomes and health care delivery. J Clin Oncol. 2018;36:2088–2100.

20. Nekhlyudov L, Mollica MA, Jacobsen PB, et al. Developing a quality of cancer survivorship care framework: Implications for clinical care, research, and policy. J Natl Cancer Inst. 2019;111:1120–1130.

21. Mollica MA, McWhirter G, Tonorezos E, et al. Developing national cancer survivorship standards to inform quality of care in the United States using a consensus approach. J Cancer Surviv. 2024;18:1190–1199.

22. Lisy K, Ly L, Kelly H, et al. How do we define and measure optimal care for cancer survivors? An online modified reactive delphi study. Cancers (Basel). 2021;13.

23. Moloczij N, Krishnasamy M, Butow P, et al. Barriers and facilitators to the implementation of audio-recordings and question prompt lists in cancer care consultations: A qualitative study. Patient Educ Couns. 2017;100:1083–1091.

Further Reading and Resources

American College of Surgeons Commission on Cancer. Optimal resources for cancer care (2020 standards). Updated December 2024. https://accreditat ion.facs.org/accreditationdocuments/CoC/Standards/Optimal_Resour ces_for_Cancer_Care.pdf

American Society of Clinical Oncology. Survivorship compendium. https://www. asco.org/news-initiatives/current-initiatives/cancer-care-initiatives/prevent ion-survivorship/survivorship-compendium. Accessed Feb 1 2025.

Australian Cancer Survivorship Centre. www.petermac.org/cancersurvivorship. Accessed Feb 1 2025.

National Cancer Institute, Office of Cancer Survivorship. National standards for cancer survivorship care toolkit. 2024. https://cancercontrol.cancer.gov/ sites/default/files/2024-10/DCCPS_National_Cancer_Survivorship_Standa rds_Toolkit_508.pdf

National Comprehensive Cancer Network. NCCN Clinical Practice Guidelines in Oncology (NCCN Guidelines). Survivorship. Version 2.2024. https://www. nccn.org/guidelines/guidelines-detail?category=3&id=1466

Nekhlyudov L, Bellizzi K, Galligan A, King-Kallimanis B, Mayer DK, Miaskowski C, Salz T, McCarty C, Cox L, Hill C, Hendershot TP, Maiese DR, Hamilton CM. The PhenX Toolkit: Standard measurement resources for cancer outcomes and survivorship research. J Natl Cancer Inst. 2023 Apr 11;115(4):473–476. doi: 10.1093/jnci/djad010.

NHS England and NHS Improvement. Living with and beyond cancer. Implementing personalised stratified follow up pathways. A handbook for local health and care systems. 2020. Publishing Approval Reference: 000889. https://www. england.nhs.uk/publication/implementing-personalised-stratified-follow-up- pathways/

NHS Improvement. Innovation to implementation: Stratified pathways of care for people living with or beyond cancer – A "how to guide." 2016. https://www. england.nhs.uk/publication/innovation-to-implementation-stratified-pathw ays-of-care-for-people-living-with-or-beyond-cancer-a-how-to-guide/

Peter MacCallum Cancer Centre. Questions you may wish to ask about the time after treatment. https://www.petermac.org/component/edocman/acsc- fact-sheet-question-prompt-sheet-060421/viewdocument/159?Itemid=0

Peter MacCallum Cancer Centre. Victorian Quality Cancer Survivorship Care Framework and Policy Template. 2021. https://www.petermac.org/patients- and-carers/support-and-wellbeing/life-after-treatment/survivorship/victor ian-quality-cancer-survivorship-care-framework

Chapter 2

Anxiety and Adjustment Disorders

Alex King, Anja Mehnert-Theuerkauf, and Daniel McFarland

Learning Objectives

After reading this chapter, the clinician will be able to:

1. Evaluate patients struggling to adapt to cancer survivorship who may suffer from an underlying anxiety or adjustment disorder.
2. Understand the prevalence of adjustment and anxiety disorders in survivorship and their clinical implications.
3. Incorporate theoretical models (e.g., psychological distress, stress and coping, general adaptation, and physiological feedback mechanisms) to explain symptomatology.
4. Approach anxiety reduction using psychopharmacology and psychological modalities in cancer survivors.
5. Facilitate psychological adaptation to a "new" normal in cancer survivorship.
6. Understand professional issues linked to management of anxiety disorders.

Background Evidence

Psychological distress can be adaptive and functional or nonadaptive and dysfunctional.[1] Therefore, distress can be operationalized to screen for maladaptive psychological states such as adjustment and anxiety disorders. Most patients with anxiety disorders experience distress, making it an ideal nonstigmatizing screening metric. The National Comprehensive Cancer Network (NCCN) publishes Distress Screening guidelines, which should be implemented in survivorship. They identify patients who stand to benefit from psychological care and who would otherwise not seek it out.

Understandably, many patients are compelled to prioritize cancer treatment and physical well-being and may not even realize the ways in which poor mental health can undermine all aspects of health and survivorship. For example, patients who have completed cancer treatment often wish to reestablish their pre-cancer lives only to find that the experience makes that impossible and this precipitates psychological distress.

This inclusive concept captures patients who are struggling to adapt or who continue to suffer from the indelible mark cancer leaves on patients' lives. It normalizes and validates commonly experienced emotions in the resilient while identifying those patients with clinically significant anxiety. Without a screening tool or extremely inquisitive and understanding clinicians, a pathological state of anxiety can easily be overlooked by clinicians who consider it a normal reaction.

Clinically Significant Anxiety and Adjustment Disorders

For some patients, the intensity, persistence, and functional impact of distress will reach thresholds for clinically significant disorders. Descriptive studies that use different measures of anxiety provide a range of distress and anxiety prevalence across cancer types and clinical settings. In cancer survivorship, the prevalence of any psychiatric disorder is elevated compared to the general population. Between 12.5% and 41% of cancer survivors experience long-term mental health difficulties.[1] Young adult cancer survivors exhibit an even higher likelihood of experiencing mental health problems. Depression, anxiety, and stress-related disorders are common psychiatric comorbidities in long-term cancer survivors. Specifically, adjustment and anxiety disorders range from a prevalence of 10% to 30%. In a robust meta-analysis by Mitchell and colleagues that pooled data from 94 studies and 14,000 patients, the prevalence of anxiety disorder was calculated at 15% and adjustment disorder at 19.4% in oncology/hematology settings, and 9.8% and 15.4%, respectively, in palliative care settings.[2] The authors suggested a 30–40% prevalence of any mood complication in the first 5 years after diagnosis, measured by clinical interview, taking into account the relative overlap of adjustment and mood disorders.[2]

Compared with the age- and sex-adjusted general population, people affected by cancer show a 2.7-fold increased risk of anxiety.[3] Patients participating in cancer rehabilitation displayed a higher prevalence of anxiety.[3] A synthesis of the literature on trajectories of multiple forms of clinically significant distress including anxiety could not derive confident conclusions about factors predicting persistence (e.g., age, income, or education) although pre-existing anxiety diagnoses, intrusive physical symptoms, and general health function are potentially relevant.[4]

Walker and colleagues reviewed the data for low- and lower-middle-income countries (LLMIC) and concluded that the prevalence of depression and anxiety appears to be increased compared to upper-income countries. Many of the review papers considered note the lack of representation of LLMIC populations in studies and datasets, and therefore extrapolations should be cautious.[5]

General Adjustment Model

A general process model as described by Brennan and colleagues presents adjustment as a continuous, iterative, and nondeterministic process.[6] At every point in the cancer "journey," what the person experiences in reality can disconfirm their implicit mental models of safety, control, identity, and the future, resulting in mental distress and disorganization. Given time and sufficient coping resources, the person will typically process and acclimate to these new experiences to form revised mental models that can better regulate emotion and guide effective action in the new reality. The clinical utility of this model is in normalizing that distress is subjective and nonlinear; that the focus should be on inputs to support the person to stabilize, reflect, learn, and adapt; and that there is no expectation of a "return to baseline," rather pointing out that a "new normal" will gradually be formed.[7,8]

Theoretical Models for Anxiety in Cancer

A Biological Perspective

The general stress response provides a framework for understanding the somatic components of anxiety. The biological underpinning of stress goes beyond the fight-or-flight response that enables us to avoid danger. It provides the biological substrate from which our bodies can face adversity for a sustained period by activating the hypothalamic-pituitary-adrenal (HPA) axis. Feedback mechanisms allow the HPA axis to be turned on and off. However, misinterpretation of threat can override the system, effectively shutting down the negative feedback loop. The HPA axis begins with corticotrophin-releasing factor synthesis and secretion leading to the production of glucocorticoid. Patients with cancer often have increased peripheral inflammation from cancer-related tissue damage and anticancer therapies along with other sources of chronic inflammation (e.g., tobacco use, obesity). Excessive chronic inflammation decreases negative feedback responsiveness to glucocorticoids. This derangement of an unregulated stress response contributes to the perpetuation of anxiety and heightened emotional reactivity.[9] In addition, the downregulation of gamma-aminobutyric acid (GABA), the primary inhibitory neurotransmitter in the brain, also perpetuates anxiety and emotional dysregulation. GABA regulates nervous system activity by mediating the flow of information between neurons. Anxiolytic medications like benzodiazepines work by activating GABA receptors and restoring the inhibitory neurotransmitter function.

A Psychological Perspective

In the 1980s, Lazarus and Folkman established the transactional model of stress and coping, the keystone of understanding how people adapt to stressors. This model is parsimonious and flexible. It posits that the psychological response to each stressor is determined by the individual's automatic, subjective appraisal of the stressor (i.e., "What does this mean for me?") combined with their subjective sense of resilience, strengths, and vulnerabilities (i.e., "Do I have the resources to manage this?").[10] Applied to cancer, stressors can be wide-ranging, from acknowledging the cancer diagnosis itself; to emerging symptoms and physical ramifications; to dealing with healthcare system demands, financial constraints, and its social implications. Each of these can have different subjective threat and coping appraisals, resulting in very individual patterns of stress even within a narrow objective category (e.g., patients receive news of their cancer stage).

Building upon Lazarus and Folkman, Curran and colleagues presented an integrated model that combined multiple theoretical models to propose a detailed framework for the development and maintenance of anxiety in the context of cancer[11] (see Figure 2.1). The relevant concepts include vulnerability factors (e.g., pre-existing schemas), the inherently uncertain and intrusive nature of cancer, subjective beliefs about the threat of cancer, cognitive processes (e.g., hypervigilance), coping responses (e.g., overcontrol), and contextual factors (e.g., subjective sense of safety in relation to one's healthcare team, social roles, and social support). The authors suggested that, in clinical practice, the model particularly directs attention to the person's beliefs about death and cancer outlook, their tolerance of uncertainty, excessive control behavior, and social communication patterns.

Presenting Problems

As an emotion, anxiety engenders an uneasy feeling of tension and physical discomfort like muscle tension and perspiration, along with troublesome worrying thoughts. Anxiety is a nonspecific feeling of an enduring diffuse threat leading to apprehension about the future, whereas fear is more consistent with a short-lived, appropriate reaction to a present and easily identifiable threat. Although the two concepts are often used interchangeably, an appreciation of their overlapping qualities and distinct differences has diagnostic implications. Adverse psychological outcomes are generally tied to anxiety rather than fear, which is often adaptive and can remit over time. Pathological adjustment and anxiety disorders indicate suffering beyond an expected response and loss of executive function in one or more key personal domains (e.g., interpersonal or occupational problems). In the survivorship context, anxiety may impact decisional capacity and perception of disease-related and other decisions, adherence to medications, cancer screening and surveillance, adaptive coping strategies, and health-related quality of life (HRQOL).

Adjustment disorders are tied to the causal stressor event. They are listed in *Diagnostic and Statistical Manual of Mental Disorders* (DSM-5R) under "Trauma- and Stressor-Related Disorders" (e.g., PTSD) but share many of the same anxiety symptoms seen in other anxiety disorders.

Table 2.1 shows common physical and psychological anxiety symptoms. It demonstrates the overlap of interconnected physical and psychological symptoms as part of all anxiety disorders. A marked vegetative response characterized by feeling uneasy is followed by an emotional/cognitive response that may precipitate motoric action (i.e., wish to fight or flee).

- *Generalized anxiety disorder*. Characterized by excessive anxiety and worry about a variety of topics for at least 6 months. The worry is difficult to control and is associated with restlessness, feeling on edge, difficulty concentrating, irritability, muscle tension, and sleep disturbance.
- *Panic disorder*. Characterized by recurrent panic attacks, which are discrete periods of intense physical and psychological discomfort (e.g., breathlessness, perspiration, doomsday feeling) that develop quickly, peaking within

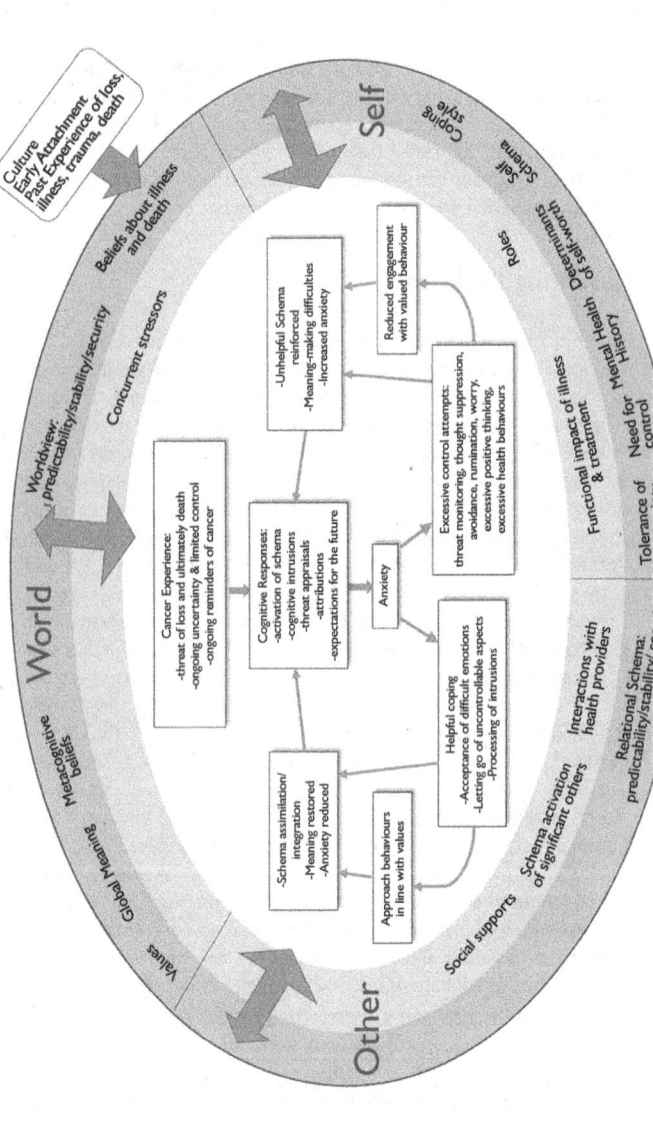

Figure 2.1 Model of interacting schemas of self and others in the world to generate coping with anxiety outcomes in cancer care.

Table 2.1 Common physical and psychological anxiety symptoms

Typical physical symptoms	Typical psychological symptoms
Increased heart rate, palpitations (tachycardia)	Feelings of anxiety and/or fear
	Fear of losing control
Faintness, feelings of dizziness	Fear of going crazy
Shortness of breath	Fear of dying
Sweating	Feelings of unreality, numbness
Feeling of tightness of the chest	Catastrophizing thoughts
Light-headedness	Constant brooding
Sensations of (abdominal) discomfort	Worries about future, treatments, side effects
Nausea, loss of appetite, diarrhea, vomiting	
	Nervousness
Inner tension, motor tension, tremor	Concentration problems
Irritability	Fear of recurrence or progression

minutes. At least one attack must be followed by a month of persistent worry about having another attack.

- *Agoraphobia.* Fear of situations where escape might be difficult or embarrassing, often comorbid with panic disorder (e.g., MRI scanner).
- *Specific phobia.* Persistent fear of an object or situation (e.g., phlebotomy or invasive procedures) that causes significant distress, impairment, or avoidance.
- *Substance/medication-induced anxiety disorder.* Etiology is directly tied to medication (e.g., corticosteroids) or substance (e.g., caffeine, cannabis, alcohol) characterized by tremor, anxiety, or panic attacks and not better explained by another anxiety disorder.
- *Anxiety disorder due to another medical condition.* Same as above, with panic attacks or anxiety but with evidence from history, physical examination, or laboratory findings relating symptoms to medical condition (e.g., hyperthyroidism, hyponatremia, Addison disease).
- *Trauma- and stressor-related disorders.* This spectrum of reactive disease states spans from the commonly diagnosed adjustment disorders (AD) to acute stress (ASD) and post-traumatic stress (PTSD) disorders. Marked distress out of proportion to the stressor, ruling out other psychiatric disorders, and functional impairment are required to meet criteria for AD with anxiety, but other subtypes include the presence of depressed mood, mixed anxiety/depression, disturbance of emotion and/or conduct, or unspecified.

ASD and PTSD are surprisingly rare in cancer populations given the refinement of diagnostic criteria that delineate the circumstances under which a cancer diagnosis or treatment can be considered a traumatic event, an issue that continues to be debated in research literature. DSM-5R criteria allow PTSD to be diagnosed only when there has been a sudden, catastrophic event *in addition* to the cancer diagnosis (e.g., life-threatening hemorrhage).

Esser and colleagues performed diagnostic interviews on 2,141 patients with all cancer types and found any-event PTSD over the course of a year was 5%.[12] The authors noted that while PTSD is rarely the correct diagnostic category, 77% of people had experienced at least one potentially lifetime traumatic event, thus potentiating cancer-related trauma, and 30% reported severe distress.

• *Obsessive-compulsive disorder*. Of note, anxiety is a key feature of obsessive-compulsive disorder (OCD) and related disorders (e.g., hoarding, body dysmorphic disorder) in addition to other affective (e.g., major depression), neurocognitive (delirium or dementia), and psychotic (e.g., schizoaffective) disorders. Anxiety may accompany any psychiatric disorder (e.g., demoralization, dissociative or personality disorders) even when the clinical presentation emphasizes other pathological aspects of illness.

Investigations for Key Differential Diagnoses

A biopsychosocial assessment should yield a differential diagnosis of cancer-related anxiety and clarify its etiology while elucidating the overlap with post-cancer (treatment)–related symptoms.

Biophysical Factors

Physical sequelae are common following cancer treatments (e.g., chemotherapy, immunotherapy, radiation, and surgery). For example, many chemotherapeutic agents affect cardiovascular function. Table 2.1 demonstrates physical conditions by organ system and associated psychological symptomatology.

In addition, clinicians should be wary of medication-induced anxiety symptoms. Cancer treatment may impair liver and renal function, which impact the body's ability to metabolize medications, which is particularly problematic for older patients on multiple medications. Those using alcohol and illicit substances may similarly experience impaired metabolism. Clinicians should consider not only the consequences of direct medication effects but also withdrawal symptoms and the effects of long-term medication use (e.g., secondary adrenal insufficiency from prolonged corticosteroid use, withdrawal from selective serotonin reuptake inhibitors [SSRIs] or benzodiazepines). Antiemetic or cachexia medications with antidopaminergic activity (e.g., prochlorperazine, metoclopramide, or olanzapine) may cause apathy or amotivational states in addition to tardive dyskinesia. Compromised lung function (e.g., pneumonitis) and hypoxia may lead to encephalopathy and anxiety. Post-cancer treatment fatigue or bone marrow failure syndromes exacerbate psychiatric symptoms. Head and neck cancer treatments, such as surgery and radiation along with small molecule inhibitor medications like tyrosine kinase inhibitors or immunotherapy, can affect thyroid function acutely or on a long-term basis.

Psychosocial Factors

The process of developing a psychosocial formulation will be most robust when it systematically follows an evidence-based theoretical model, such as the integrated model.[11] Clinicians should explore vulnerability factors (e.g., pre-existing schemas), subjective beliefs about the threat of cancer, cognitive processes (e.g., hypervigilance), coping responses (e.g., overcontrol), and relevant contextual factors (e.g., relationship to healthcare, social support). Collaborative formulation building and reflection with the patient is therapeutic and establishes a positive foundation for subsequent evidence-based psychosocial interventions to reduce anxiety and existential angst.

In the survivorship context, it is important to consider the widespread impact cancer has on interpersonal and occupational functioning. Patients may be experiencing newly found isolation or social rejection/withdrawal, especially when interpersonal skills and resilience do not withstand adversity. Many patients begin to process the personal meaning of the cancer diagnosis only after they have completed its treatments. Anxiety may stem from various sources.

Anxiety Types Unique to the Cancer or Survivorship Setting

Fear of Cancer Recurrence or Progression

Fear of cancer recurrence (FCR) and fear of cancer progression (FCP) are dealt with extensively in Chapter 3. This fear, while specific and counterproductive, is also free-floating and more akin to anxiety in general. It is frequently accompanied by somatization. Luigjes-Huizer and colleagues identified that 19% of patients self-report very high FCR, while 59% report at least a moderate level.[13] FCR occurs across cancer types and stages of survivorship, with women and younger patients more likely to report greater FCR.

"Scanxiety" or "Markeritis"

Cancer surveillance is stressful. Some patients only have significant distress or anxiety around the time of testing to determine the possibility of recurrence. This symptom compartmentalization is understandable given the perceived risk but may occur alongside other forms of anxiety. Patients may worry about getting the procedure itself (e.g., scan, phlebotomy), what the results reveal, or having to endure waiting until they are discussed.

Existential/Death Anxiety

Most patients with cancer experience preoccupation with mortality, but a significant minority experience an intense fear of death or the dying process. A study found that 32% of patients with cancer experienced moderate to severe death anxiety.[14] While the concern is higher in patients with advanced cancer, it also affects patients with no evidence of disease.

Anxiety and Psychopathology in Relatives and Caregivers

Cancer affects the entire family unit or social circle, often requiring significant care and attention to the mental health of those around the patient who are also processing a loss. Almost half of caregivers experience significant anxiety while up to 40% experience depressive symptoms in addition to loneliness, demoralization, and grief.[15] Caregivers' mental health directly affects patients with cancer (see also Chapter 6).

Safety Assessment

Although major depression is strongly linked to suicide, depressed patients with a comorbid anxiety disorder or agitation are even more likely to commit suicide. While the true rate of suicides is likely underreported and the absolute number remains low (twice the general population), patients with cancer commit suicide at much higher rates (15 times the general population) immediately following diagnosis or recurrence (weeks or months).[16] Therefore, addressing adjustment and anxiety at these time points is essential since recurrence can happen throughout survivorship. Other high-risk factors include impulsiveness, drug and alcohol overuse, neurodiversity, persistent pain, recent loss, poor prognosis or recurrence, healthcare avoidance, and high symptom burden.

Psychometric Assessment

Validated screening tools and clinician-rated or self-report questionnaires complement the clinical evaluations of psychological symptoms. They provide consistency in measuring symptoms longitudinally. Table 2.2 provides examples.

Table 2.2 Measures of anxiety and related symptoms validated in cancer settings	
Anxiety scale	**Description**
The Distress Thermometer and Problem List	One-item, nondiagnostic tool measures distress and associated problems. Endorsed by the National Comprehensive Cancer Network (NCCN) for mandated screening
Generalized Anxiety Disorder-7 (GAD-7)	Brief seven-item measure frequently used in cancer settings meant to evaluate generalized anxiety disorder. ≥10 screens in anxiety (screening) while 5, 10, and 15 = mild, moderate, and severe anxiety levels, respectively.
Hospital Anxiety and Depression Scale (HADS)	Legacy measure of anxiety and depression in somatically ill patients. 0–7 = normal; 8–10 = possible/borderline anxiety or depressive disorder; ≥11 = probable anxiety or depressive disorder.
Patient-Reported Outcomes Measurement Information System (PROMIS®)	Self-report measure derived from legacy measure and can be compared across various psychosocial domains. PROMIS-anxiety has multiple forms (short or full length; computer adapted).
Fear of Cancer Recurrence Inventory (FCRI)	Measures FCR in research and clinical domains. 42-item measure but also comes in 9-item short form [FCRI-SF]
Death and Dying Distress Scale (DADDS)	Two-factor measure: (1) "Finitude of life" and (2) "Death-related distress"

Clinical Management

Pharmacologic Treatments

Pharmacologic treatment is warranted for patients with moderate to severe anxiety disorders to ameliorate symptoms and restore psychosocial functioning. Antidepressants, mood stabilizers, benzodiazepines, neuroleptics, and adjunctive agents (e.g., beta-blockers) play a key role in cancer survivorship rehabilitation. The first-line agents include ##SSRIs, atypical antidepressants, and, to a lesser extent, serotonin norepinephrine reuptake inhibitors (SNRIs) (see Table 2.3). Patients should be counseled on indications, expectations (i.e., benefit within 2–6 weeks), and side-effect profiles and encouraged to use the lowest effective dose. Depending on the risk (e.g., previous suicide attempts), severity of disease, and patient preferences, the duration of treatment should parallel the natural illness trajectory (typically 9–12 months) or longer. Benzodiazepines are mild tranquilizing medications with immediate efficacy and the potential for physiological dependence, and they should be prescribed and deprescribed thoughtfully while favoring other non–habit-forming agents.

While medication efficacy matters, the choice of agent (e.g., SSRI or SNRI) depends mostly on its side-effect profile to maximize benefit (e.g., using a sedating agent in a patient with insomnia), noted personal or familial benefit from and tolerability to an agent, patient preference, and availability (e.g., cost). Some side effects are to be avoided (e.g., sexual) while others may be clinically beneficial (e.g., sedation, weight gain). Table 2.3 highlights some considerations to maximizing medication benefit.

Psychological Therapies

Patients in the survivorship setting have many interrelated psychosocial needs that require a comprehensive approach. Social, occupational, and financial adjustment assumes an important role in the post-cancer treatment setting. Patients find themselves making various lifestyle changes such as cessation of smoking and substance misuse, losing an important social support system at the cancer center, or physical limitations. Collaborative agenda setting as part of a psychosocial assessment helps establish rapport and validates patients' emotions and experiences. Caregivers may play an integral role in psychosocial adjustment, especially because patients suffering from anxiety disorders may not appreciate the broader perspective cancer has played in their lives. Patients may be particularly sensitive to social cues that they feel are invalidating, stigmatizing, or intrusive. They may be ambivalent about engaging with psychosocial care; therefore, the task of establishing transparency and collaboration is particularly significant. Therapeutic modalities are delivered in various formats; individual, group, digital or tele-based, or collaborative care model–based therapies are efficacious.

Psychotherapy and psychopharmacology are comparable in terms of their efficacy, but psychotropics should not be used alone because there is much more to be gained by their combined use. Moreover, combinatory therapy has distinct advantages (medication may allow for more focused or intensive psychotherapy). Choice of psychotherapy varies based on anxiety disorder

Table 2.3 Examples of pharmacologic agents to address anxiety disorders in the survivorship setting.

Medication	Dose range (mg)	FDA approved	Off-label uses	Comments
Selective serotonin reuptake inhibitors (SSRIs)				
Escitalopram	10–20	GAD	PD, SAD	Limited DDI, weak 2D6 metabolism and used with tamoxifen and abiraterone
Sertraline	50–200	PD, SAD	GAD	Highest sexual SE, moderate 2D6, competes with tamoxifen and abiraterone
Fluoxetine	20–60	PD	GAD, PD, SAD	Long half-life, high 2D6 metabolism
Paroxetine	20–60	GAD, PD, SAD	-	Sedating, high 2D6 metabolism decreases tamoxifen and abiraterone efficacy, withdrawal SE
Atypical agents				
Mirtazapine	15–90	-	Anxiety, GAD, PD, SAD	Helps insomnia, nausea, anorexia
Buspirone	15–60	Anxiety	GAD	Used adjunctively, may lessen SSRI-induced sexual SE
Hydroxyzine	25–100	Anxiety	GAD, PD, SAD	Sedating, non–habit-forming
Serotonin norepinephrine reuptake inhibitors (SNRIs)				
Duloxetine	30–120	GAD	PD, SAD	Indicated for peripheral neuropathy, co-analgesic with neuropathic pain
Venlafaxine	75–300	GAD	PD, SAD	Treats hot flashes, co-analgesic, withdrawal SE
Benzodiazepines				
Alprazolam	1–2	Anxiety, PD	GAD, PD, SAD	Useful to abort panic attacks, prominent dependence
Clonazepam	1–4	PD	Anxiety, GAD, PD, SAD	Long half-life, restless legs, anticonvulsant

Table 2.3 Continued

Medication	Dose range (mg)	FDA approved	Off-label uses	Comments
Lorazepam	1–6	Anxiety	GAD, PD, SAD	Limited DDI, safest with liver disease
GABAergic				
Pregabalin	150–600	–	GAD, SAD	Indicated for fibromyalgia and neuropathic pain
Gabapentin	600–2,400	–	GAD, SAD, PD	Adjunctive pain treatment
Neuroleptics				
Olanzapine	2.5–15	–	Anxiety, GAD	Indicated for chemotherapy-induced nausea and cachexia; insomnia induced by dexamethasone
Quetiapine	25–300	–	Anxiety, GAD	Sedating, useful hypnotic, steroid-induced insomnia

Abbreviations: DDI, drug-drug interaction; FDA, US Food and Drug Administration; GAD, generalized anxiety disorder; PD, panic disorder; SAD, social anxiety disorder; SE, side effects; SSRI, selective serotonin reuptake inhibitor

Source: Garakani A, Murrough JW, Freire RC, et al. Pharmacotherapy of anxiety disorders: Current and emerging treatment options. Front Psychiatry. 2020;11:595584. doi: 10.3389/fpsyt.2020.59558417

type, severity, and patient preference.[18] Early diagnosis and treatment improve outcomes and reduce the burden of these diseases.

Psychoeducation

Psychoeducation parallels the process of patient-centered learning in oncology and facilitates the adjustment to mental health challenges and the integration of selfhood that is integral to survivorship coping.[19] Education can accompany other modalities like problem-solving or supportive-expressive therapy.

Cognitive Behavioral Therapy

Cognitive behavioral therapy (CBT) is the most widely evaluated time-limited modality and has proven efficacy in many psychopathological settings and is highly adaptable. CBT entails behavioral activation, identifying and challenging negative thought patterns and behaviors, and replacing cognitive distortions and perceptual limitations with adaptive and expansive alternatives. The therapeutic approach encompasses cognitive restructuring, exposure, and response prevention techniques.

Mindfulness-Based Therapies

Many mind–body modalities like yoga and meditation incorporate mindfulness, but manualized approaches demonstrate efficacy that appropriately addresses anxiety disorders. Mindfulness-based stress reduction (MBSR) focuses on increasing awareness of the present moment and reducing rumination about negative thoughts. It can be delivered individually or through groups.

Acceptance Commitment Therapy

Acceptance commitment therapy (ACT) incorporates mindfulness-based behavior therapy to help patients develop psychological flexibility by accepting their thoughts and feelings without judgment and committing to actions aligned with their personal values. Participants are taught to embrace the present, take meaningful action, and engage with difficult emotions.

Meaning-Centered Psychotherapy and Existential Psychotherapy

These modalities are used expressly to address the existential dread, angst, or terror that may occur along the cancer survivorship continuum. They are relational, manualized, and broadly applicable for individual or group settings.

Case Study

A year ago, a woman in her late forties received all the appropriate care for a locally advanced breast cancer while remaining on an antiestrogen agent. Although she had returned to work, she was unable to concentrate because she felt "on edge" and endorsed several self-described panic attacks, all of which were highly unusual for her. She is usually calm and level-headed. She reports tolerating her antihormonal drug and is perplexed by why she's not feeling better having completed surgery, chemotherapy, and radiation treatments. She feels plagued with anxious thoughts and questions her self-worth. She denies depression and can enjoy usual activities but finds that she is much more emotionally labile than usual, is not sleeping or eating well, and struggles to keep up with her responsibilities and relationships.

She begins working with a therapist who is concerned that she has developed an anxiety disorder such as GAD or panic disorder but notes that she declares no fear of recurrence and yet eventually finds that worry about cancer recurrence and difficult feelings about what she endured in her breast cancer treatment are at the root of her anxiety symptoms. The therapist helps the patient revisit and validate her appropriate concerns around what she experienced (i.e., existential dread, difficult interpersonal strain during her cancer treatment). Psychoeducation helps her understand her anxiety response while the incorporation of ACT-based therapy provides the patient with much needed insight into how to live beyond the cancer experience; this ultimately relieves her anxiety symptoms.

This case illustrates how psychotherapy can build insight into underlying fears that contribute to the development of an anxiety disorder, and, with help, these fears can be ameliorated to enhance quality of life.

Professional Issues and Service Implementation

Recording and Communicating

Clinicians working with patients experiencing anxiety in survivorship require a broad knowledge base, self-awareness, and respect for interpersonal boundaries, all of which are facilitated by communicating and working within a multidisciplinary team.

Cultural Issues

Culturally shaped beliefs about anxiety and adjustment should be incorporated into the clinician's approach alongside a respectful and curious attitude (e.g., Is anxiety seen as "normal," "weakness," a lack of "faith," or a "neurochemical imbalance"?). Culturally discordant clinician–patient relationships require even more self-reflection upon one's beliefs, worldview positioning, and underlying assumptions as they relate to approaching the patient.

Common Ethical Dilemmas

Psychological safety is imperative and should be deliberately established to counteract any latent feelings of disempowerment and alienation in survivorship. Respect for individual differences is critical; clinicians must strive for person-centered care.

Policies for Clinical Services

Psycho-oncology professionals are well positioned to lead in developing and sustaining compassionate, trauma-informed cancer services. Psycho-oncology is integral to survivorship care and a basic human right.

Teams and Supervision

The psychosocial care team embraces the disciplines of psychology, social work, psychiatry, nursing, pastoral care, and occupational and physical therapies. Supervision ensures growth of skills and guides the development of experience in team members, beginning with trainees and extending as experience grows.

References

1. Mehnert-Theuerkauf A, Hufeld JM, Esser P, et al. Prevalence of mental disorders, psychosocial distress, and perceived need for psychosocial support in cancer patients and their relatives stratified by biopsychosocial factors: Rationale, study design, and methods of a prospective multi-center observational cohort study (LUPE study). Front Psychol. 2023;14:1125545. doi: 10.3389/fpsyg.2023.1125545.

2. Mitchell AJ, Chan M, Bhatti H, et al. Prevalence of depression, anxiety, and adjustment disorder in oncological, haematological, and palliative-care settings: A meta-analysis of 94 interview-based studies. Lancet Oncol. 2011.;12(2):160–174. doi: 10.1016/S1470-2045(11)70002-X.

3. Goerling U, Hinz A, Koch-Gromus U, Hufeld JM, Esser P, Mehnert-Theuerkauf A. Prevalence and severity of anxiety in cancer patients: Results from a multicenter cohort study in Germany. J Cancer Res Clin Oncol. 2023;149(9):6371–6379. doi: 10.1007/s00432-023-04600-w.

4. Curran L, Mahoney A, Hastings B. A systematic review of trajectories of clinically relevant distress amongst adults with cancer: Course and predictors. J Clin Psychol Med Settings. 2025;32(1):1–18. doi: 10.1007/s10880-024-10011-x.

5. Walker ZJ, Xue S, Jones MP, Ravindran AV. Depression, anxiety, and other mental disorders in patients with cancer in low- and lower-middle-income countries: A systematic review and meta-analysis. JCO Glob Oncol. 2021;7:1233–1250. doi: 10.1200/GO.21.00056.

6. Brennan J. Adjustment to cancer: Coping or personal transition? Psycho-Oncology. 2001;10(1):1–18. doi: 10.1002/1099-1611(200101/02)10:1<1::aid-pon484>3.0.co;2-t.

7. Evans C, Saliba-Serre B, Preau M, et al. Post-traumatic growth 5 years after cancer: Identification of associated actionable factors. Support Care Cancer. 2022;30(10):8261–8270. doi: 10.1007/s00520-022-07253-6.

8. Casellas-Grau A, Ochoa C, Ruini C. Psychological and clinical correlates of posttraumatic growth in cancer: A systematic and critical review. Psycho-Oncology. 2017;26(12):2007–2018. doi: 10.1002/pon.4426.

9. Haroon E, Miller AH, Sanacora G. Inflammation, glutamate, and glia: A trio of trouble in mood disorders. Neuropsychopharmacology. 2017;42(1):193–215. doi: 10.1038/npp.2016.199.

10. Lazarus RS, and Folkman, S. *Stress, Appraisal, and Coping.* New York: Springer; 1984.

11. Curran L, Sharpe L, Butow P. Anxiety in the context of cancer: A systematic review and development of an integrated model. Clin Psychol Rev. 2017;56:40–54. doi: 10.1016/j.cpr.2017.06.003.

12. Esser P, Glaesmer H, Faller H, et al. Posttraumatic stress disorder among cancer patients: Findings from a large and representative interview-based study in Germany. Psycho-Oncology. 2019;28(6):1278–1285. doi: 10.1002/pon.5079.

13. Luigjes-Huizer YL, Tauber NM, Humphris G, et al. What is the prevalence of fear of cancer recurrence in cancer survivors and patients? A systematic review and individual participant data meta-analysis. Psycho-Oncology. 2022;31(6):879–892. doi: 10.1002/pon.5921.

14. Neel C, Lo C, Rydall A, Hales S, Rodin G. Determinants of death anxiety in patients with advanced cancer. BMJ Support Palliat Care. 2015;5(4):373–380. doi: 10.1136/bmjspcare-2012-000420.

15. Sklenarova H, Krumpelmann A, Haun MW, et al. When do we need to care about the caregiver? Supportive care needs, anxiety, and depression among informal caregivers of patients with cancer and cancer survivors. Cancer. 2015;121(9):1513–1519. doi: 10.1002/cncr.29223.

16. McFarland DC, Walsh L, Napolitano S, Morita J, Jaiswal R. Suicide in patients with cancer: Identifying the risk factors. Oncology. 2019;33(6):221–226.

17. Garakani A, Murrough JW, Freire RC, et al. Pharmacotherapy of anxiety disorders: Current and emerging treatment options. Front Psychiatry. 2020;11:595584. doi: 10.3389/fpsyt.2020.595584.

18. Strohle A, Gensichen J, Domschke K. The diagnosis and treatment of anxiety disorders. Dtsch Arztebl Int. 2018;155(37):611–620. doi: 10.3238/arztebl.2018.0611.

19. Sarkhel S, Singh OP, Arora M. Clinical practice guidelines for psychoeducation in psychiatric disorders general principles of psychoeducation. Indian J Psychiatry. 2020;62(Suppl 2):S319–S323. doi: 10.4103/psychiatry.IndianJPsychiatry_780_19.

Further Reading and Resources

Breitbart WS, et al. Adjustment disorders in cancer. In: Breitbart W, et al., eds. *Psycho-Oncology*, 4th ed. Oxford University Press; 2021. Online edition: Oxford Academic, 2021. https://doi.org/10.1093/med/9780190097653.003.0041. Accessed July 31, 2025.

Grassi L, Caruso R, Riba MB, et al. ESMO Guidelines Committee. Anxiety and depression in adult cancer patients: ESMO Clinical Practice Guideline. ESMO Open. 2023;8(2):101155. doi: 10.1016/j.esmoop.2023.101155. Epub 2023 Mar 14. PMID: 37087199; PMCID: PMC10163167.

Grassi L, Nanni MG, Rodin G, Li M, Caruso R. The use of antidepressants in oncology: A review and practical tips for oncologists. Ann Oncology. 2018;29(1):101–111. doi: 10.1093/annonc/mdx526.

Teo I, Krishnan A, Lee GL. Psychosocial interventions for advanced cancer patients: A systematic review. Psycho-Oncology. 2019;28(7):1394–1407. doi: 10.1002/pon.5103.

Chapter 3

Fear of Cancer Recurrence

Sophie Lebel, Ben Smith, and Gozde Ozakinci

Learning Objectives

After reading this chapter, the clinician will be able to:

1. Understand what fear of cancer recurrence is and how it is conceptualized.
2. Have awareness of tools for its assessment in clinical practice and research.
3. Consider the psychological support options that show evidence in different healthcare systems globally.
4. Appreciate ethical, cultural, and professional issues regarding the implementation of optimal fear of cancer recurrence care.

Background Evidence

The growing number of cancer survivors globally brings welcome news. According to *The Cancer Atlas*, in 2018, there were nearly 44 million cancer survivors diagnosed within the last 5 years across the world,[1] a number that will have increased since. However, the issues faced by individuals and family members who have been through cancer diagnosis and treatment are numerous, ranging from existential concerns such as death anxiety to financial difficulties. Early writing on life after cancer treatment referenced the "sword of Damocles that hangs over the individual and family for the rest of the person's life" stating that "a person never gets over cancer."[2 (p.1201)] See Box 3.1 for a definition of fear of cancer recurrence (FCR).

Most research on FCR has been conducted with early-stage, disease-free cancer survivors rather than people living with advanced or metastatic disease. For this latter group, the concept of fear of progression (FoP) may be more relevant than FCR. However, currently, FoP is much less studied compared to FCR. Some authors postulate that FoP and FCR are "nearly identical"; others have recently argued that they are different constructs and that FCR interventions may require adaptation to address the needs of those living with advanced or metastatic cancer.[4] Research efforts are ongoing to better distinguish these two phenomena.

Box 3.1 Defining Fear of Cancer Recurrence

Fear of cancer recurrence (FCR) is a common experience for people who have been diagnosed and treated for cancer and presents itself on a severity continuum. It is defined as "the fear, worry, or concern relating to the possibility that cancer will come back or progress.[3] (p. 3266)

The precise prevalence of FCR is hard to ascertain because of the wide range of measures that have been used to study this concern. A recent meta-analysis based on one of the most common measures of FCR, the Fear of Cancer Recurrence Inventory-Short Form (FCRI-SF), shows that 59% of survivors experience at least moderate levels of this fear and 19% report a high level of fear, which would indicate need for specialized psychological support.[5]

FCR is a multidimensional psychological phenomenon that may include emotional experiences, thoughts and beliefs about cancer and its likelihood to return, triggers in the form of physiological experiences, and coping strategies. Theoretical models have been put forward to explain how FCR emerges and what factors influence its maintenance. Lee-Jones et al. have applied Leventhal's self-regulation model of illness to the understanding of FCR.[6] With emphasis on both cognitive and emotional paths that are instigated following a threat to health, the self-regulation model allows us to understand the role of mental models of illness threats (i.e., illness perceptions or beliefs) and recurrence-related beliefs (e.g., "When it comes back, this time it will be worse") and their interactions with our emotional responses to fear of cancer coming back. The model also clearly articulates the role that symptom experience plays in triggering FCR and illness perceptions and how coping with these pathways can take various forms, from seeking healthcare provider reassurance to avoiding topics that relate to cancer.

A review of FCR theoretical models found six such perspectives and identified the role of several factors in the emergence of FCR, such as life experiences (e.g., past cancer-related losses), beliefs about cancer (e.g., "It's inevitable that cancer will come back"), beliefs about the importance of worry (e.g., metacognitions such as "If I worry about cancer recurrence, then I'll be prepared"), problematic styles of information processing (e.g., rumination, attention toward threat-related information), and lack of future planning given uncertainty, which can lead to a poor self-concept.[7] In a recent study testing a model of FCR or FoP, intrusive thoughts, perceiving the cancer experience as threatening, and meta-cognitions about cancer, as well as death anxiety predicted these fears, thus highlighting the importance of theory-driven constructs. It was also noted in this study that death anxiety was associated with FCR across the disease spectrum because participants with both early- and late-stage disease were included.[8] There is emerging evidence that death anxiety may play a more prominent role in FoP compared to FCR.[4]

It is, therefore, understandable that FCR can be related to a variety of psychological outcomes. A comprehensive review on FCR has shown that high levels of FCR are associated with higher levels of distress, anxiety, and depression and a lower quality of life.[9]

Presenting Problems

Fear of cancer recurrence exists on a spectrum from mild levels of worry that may play an adaptive role in motivating positive health behaviors through to severe/clinical FCR, which may cause significant disruption in day-to-day functioning. Table 3.1 reports the features of clinical FCR that reached expert consensus in a recent Delphi study.[10] Experts were in favor of using these criteria to indicate clinical FCR rather than applying a diagnosis from the Diagnostic and Statistical Manual of Mental Disorders (DSM-5).[11]

Higher FCR has been associated with under/overuse of health services as some patients may cope with FCR through either avoidance (i.e., trying to avoid thoughts/reminders of recurrence) or, conversely, seeking medical reassurance. These coping strategies are not part of the features of clinical FCR, but clinicians should we aware of them because they may provide short-term relief from FCR. However, they ultimately reinforce the threat of recurrence and maintain FCR in the longer term.[6]

FCR is common across people with different types of cancer, stages of disease, treatment experiences, and time post-treatment. Clinical characteristics related to objective risk of recurrence, such as cancer type or stage and treatment type or time since treatment have demonstrated limited associations with FCR.[9] However, more intensive treatment (e.g., combinations of adjuvant therapies) have been shown to predict higher FCR.[9]

🔑 Key Point
Patient/survivor FCR appears interrelated with caregiver FCR, so when high FCR is identified in one dyad member, it may be sensible to check for FCR in the other.

FCR may co-occur with other forms of psychological morbidity, such as generalized anxiety disorder, but this is not always the case. While FCR may share features with anxiety/depression, such as intrusive thoughts or rumination, it

Table 3.1 Features of clinical fear of cancer recurrence (FCR)
Clinical FCR is characterized by at least three of the following features being present for 3 months or more.
High levels of:
1. preoccupation
2. worry
3. that are persistent*
4. hypervigilance to physical symptoms.
Functional impairment may also be considered.
* Present at least 50% of the time (i.e., not just around follow-up appointments or waiting for test results).

> **Box 3.2 Factors Most Strongly Correlated with Higher Fear of Cancer Recurrence (FCR)**
>
> - Younger age
> - The presence of treatment side effects
> - Psychological comorbidities such as generalized anxiety disorder
> - Female gender
>
> It should be noted that the explanatory power of these associations is relatively limited and so it is prudent to screen for FCR in all people affected by cancer.

differs from anxiety in that the focus of worries or concerns is to some degree a rational concern. Consequently, standard cognitive behavioral therapy (CBT) approaches focused on reframing irrational fears may not be helpful in treating FCR and may even be invalidating for people with cancer who face ongoing uncertainty around recurrence.

Tools to Assess FCR

Several brief screening tools have been developed to aid rapid identification of FCR in clinical practice. Two options have the most supporting evidence:

1. *The FCR-1*, a verbal question asking, "On a scale from 0 to 100, what is your subjective level of fear of cancer recurrence at this time?" Scores ≥45 have been identified as optimal for identifying possible clinical FCR.[12]
2. *The FCR-1r* is a written question designed to be integrated into the Edmonton Symptom Assessment System (ESAS). It asks patients to rate their level of FCR on a 0–10 scale. Scores ≥5 have good sensitivity and specificity for identifying possible clinical FCR.[13]

FCR screening is particularly important given the lack of robust risk factors for FCR and that patients may be reluctant to raise their fears with their healthcare provider. Patients may not want to be seen as ungrateful for their treatment or to be questioning its efficacy. Some people may feel that FCR is something that they should be able to manage themselves. Asking about FCR in a way that normalizes it and validates peoples' experiences may help not only to identify FCR but also to encourage openness to FCR intervention and treatment (see Box 3.3).

> **Box 3.3 Example of Normalizing the Experience of FCR during a Patient Encounter**
>
> "Many people whom I see worry a lot about their cancer coming back. That's normal and expected after a cancer diagnosis. But if the worry is distressing you, or is preventing you from getting on with your life, we should do something about it. There are things we can suggest to help you manage these worries. So, has this been a problem for you?"

Investigations for Key Differential Diagnoses

Rule Out

- Thyroid disorders with assessment for goitre and thyroid function blood tests
- Anemia with FBE assessment
- Panic disorder with history of panic attacks and related physical symptoms of tremor, breathlessness, palpitations, dizziness
- Metabolic disorder with electrolytes, calcium, glucose, urea, and creatinine
- Generalized anxiety disorder and major depressive disorder

As noted above, FCR exists on a spectrum from mild, potentially adaptive levels, to clinical levels causing distress and disruption to daily life.

🔍 Key Point

Administration of a longer screening tool, such as the 9-item Fear of Cancer Recurrence Inventory – Short Form (FCRI-SF), may help differentiate the severity of FCR. While the FCRI-SF does not assess all clinical features of FCR and there is debate about cutoffs, scores 13–21/36 are widely thought to indicate moderate/subclinical FCR, while scores ≥22/36 are thought to indicate severe/clinical FCR.[14] Alternative brief tools with cutoffs to guide the characterization of FCR severity include the FCR-4/7[15] and the Cancer Worry Scale.[16]

Concurrent administration of screening tools for anxiety and depression (e.g., the GAD-7 and PHQ-9) may help differentiate whether recurrence is an isolated focus of worry and rumination, or whether it is comorbid with more generalized anxiety and/or depression. If FCR is comorbid with anxiety and/or depression, *treating these more general mental health concerns first may be warranted depending on their severity.*

In patients reporting moderate to severe FCR on screening tools, further assessment is indicated. A semi-structured interview for FCR is available for mental health specialists,[17] which is currently being updated to better capture all features of clinical FCR.[18] Non–mental health specialists may wish to ask brief questions regarding FCR triggers, persistence and impact of worries, strategies used to cope with FCR, and capacity/preference for treatment if indicated (see examples in Table 3.2). This interview may help guide the focus of treatment. For instance, in some cases, FCR may be exacerbated by uncertainty around recurrence risk and subsequent prognosis, leading to an overestimation of recurrence risk that could be addressed through information provision. In other cases, hypervigilance to symptoms and related self-examination behaviors may be exacerbating FCR, so developing a behavioral contract around self-examination frequency and more adaptive monitoring behaviors may be appropriate.

FCR may fluctuate relative to internal triggers, such as the experience of side effects, or external triggers, such as follow-up scans or appointments (FCR in this context may be referred to as "scanxiety"). Therefore, it

Table 3.2 Questions to use to assess clinical fear of cancer recurrence (FCR)

Guiding questions	Responses that might indicate clinical significance
How frequently do you have thoughts related to the cancer returning? How long do these thoughts last? Do you find these thoughts difficult to control?	Reports frequent death-related thoughts that are hard to control and that last 30 minutes or longer
Do you routinely scan or pay attention to physical sensations in your body? How often?	Reports preoccupations with physical sensations in the body, attributing pain or sensations to a recurrence
On a scale of 0 to 10, how strongly do you believe the cancer will return?	Reports a strong belief that the thoughts are true and might provide reasons to support this belief (e.g., previous misdiagnosis)
How have these thoughts or beliefs affected your life?	Might report panic, worry, stress, a need to escape, trouble sleeping, fatigue, or difficulties or uncertainty about planning for the future

is important to rescreen and assess patients at different time points (e.g., screening before a follow-up appointment, further assessment/discussion during or after) to assess the persistence of FCR, which is a key indicator of clinical significance. Rescreening or assessment of FCR is also important to capture changes in FCR in response to intervention and whether the level of intervention or support needs to be stepped up or down.

Clinical Management

Recommendations in this section are based on a published guideline around the management of FCR and based on severity level (low, moderate, high).[19] Please see Figure 3.1 for an overview of the recommendations. Healthcare teams are encouraged to consider two models of care delivery for the management of FCR: a matched-care approach (i.e., survivors are referred to services based on their level of FCR after the initial assessment) or a stepped-care approach (i.e., survivors start with lower-intensity intervention, such as information from their oncologist during a follow-up appointment, and, after reassessment of their FCR, may receive more intensive intervention).[20]

For survivors assessed to have low FCR, healthcare providers can routinely provide information around prognosis and risk of recurrence, signs and symptoms of recurrence, and what follow-up care entails (which might also be included in a survivorship care plan), along with normalization of FCR as a common issue, especially around hospital visits and waiting for test results. A systematic review of FCR interventions by non–mental health specialists found that consultation duration, empathy, and clear information delivery helped decrease FCR and concluded that the provision of honest information about prognosis and recurrence risk was helpful to address FCR.[21] Healthcare

Guideline 19–7

FCR Screening, Assessment, and Intervention Flow Chart

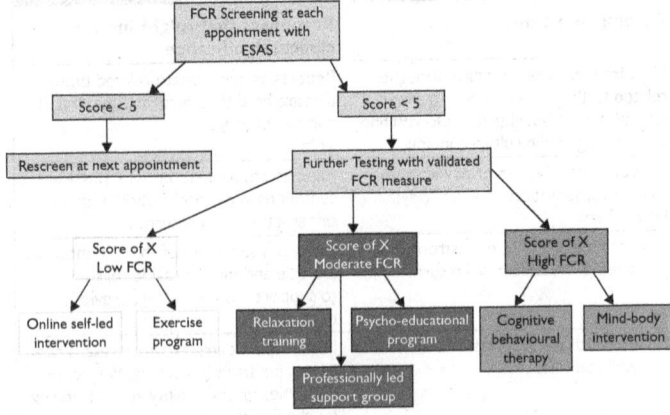

Figure 3.1 FCR screening, assessment, and intervention flow chart

Source: Lebel S, Zwaal C, Craig L, et al. Fear of Cancer Recurrence Guideline. Cancer Care Ontario. 2024. https://www.cancercareontario.ca/en/guidelines-advice/types-of-cancer/75576.

Box 3.4 Communicating Information to Reduce FCR

For everyone with FCR, regardless of severity levels, healthcare professionals are encouraged to discuss

- Prognosis and its basis.
- The most likely signs and symptoms of a recurrence (as well as those not likely to be related to cancer) and symptom intensity and duration that should prompt help-seeking.
- Recommended behaviors to reduce risk (such as smoking cessation and exercise).
- Standard follow-up schedules and their rationale.

This information could also be offered as a psychoeducation group/class.

---

providers can also recommend useful coping strategies such as engaging in self-care, talking about their fear with supportive others, journaling, and reducing stress. Healthcare providers can suggest exercise programs following recommended country-specific exercise guidelines and online or remote self-led interventions, where available. Online or remote interventions that offer guidance (by a clinician or trained personnel) may increase program engagement, satisfaction, and benefit.[19]

For survivors with moderate FCR, healthcare providers can recommend moderately intensive, general resources (Box 3.5) such as a psycho-educational class or program, relaxation training and/or a professionally led support group.[19] Preliminary evidence shows that these resources might be more effective when delivered in group format.[19] A psycho-educational class

---

Box 3.5 Helping Survivors Cope with Their FCR

1. Encourage survivors to adopt good coping strategies:
   - Engaging in enjoyed activities
   - Meditation/religion, yoga, physical activity, writing in a journal
   - Talking to family, friends, and other survivors about their fears
   - Joining a support group
2. Discourage unhelpful coping like avoidance, fatalism, or requesting additional tests.

---

or program can provide structured education about cancer and treatment management, survivorship and surveillance guidelines and information on effective ways of managing the risk of recurrence and FCR. This class or program can be delivered by a range of healthcare professionals with experience in oncology. One study found that cancer survivors with moderate FCR benefited from attending five relaxation training sessions that consisted of demonstrating and assigning as homework the practice of various forms of relaxation such as progressive muscular relaxation, deep breathing, and guided imagery.[22] Professionally led support groups that span several sessions and enable expression of emotions and meaning-making around the cancer experience may be beneficial for patients and survivors who experience moderate FCR.[19] For all the recommended moderately intensive interventions, healthcare teams are encouraged to consider existing resources within their local hospital, cancer center, and community to avoid duplication of services and facilitate implementation.

For survivors with high FCR, there is strong evidence from several systematic reviews and meta-analyses[23,24] that brief six- or seven-session high-intensity psychological interventions that directly target FCR have small to moderate effects in the short-term and that gains are maintained over time. These interventions can cost-effectively reduce FCR, improve quality of life and role functioning, and decrease psychological distress.[21]

The most researched therapeutic options include CBT (i.e., therapies that focus on the contents of thoughts and aim to identify and modify people's negative thoughts or those that help people identify their thought processes and relate to these experiences differently) and mind–body interventions (including relaxation techniques, meditation etc.).[19] These interventions can be delivered in a group or an individual format, with preliminary evidence suggesting that groups may be slightly more efficacious[23] and that third-wave CBT (e.g., mindfulness, acceptance commitment therapy [ACT]) may be more efficacious than traditional CBT that focuses on challenging thoughts.[23] They can be offered face-to-face, virtually, or in a blended format. To date, the efficacy of these interventions has been tested when they have been offered by mental health specialists (e.g., psychiatrists, psychologists, social workers, and trainees of these disciplines); their efficacy when offered by non–mental health specialists (e.g., nurses, other allied health professionals) has yet to be demonstrated.[19] Some of the most

Box 3.6 Managing Clinical FCR: Common Interventions

- Identify triggers of FCR and the emotional, physical, and behavioral manifestations of FCR.
- Provide information about signs and symptoms of recurrence to decrease hypervigilance to physical symptoms.
- Decrease less-adaptive coping strategies (e.g., Googling symptoms) and encourage new coping strategies (e.g., mindfulness meditations, attention training, or relaxation techniques).
- Help survivors to react differently to their thoughts, whether through cognitive restructuring or thought defusion/detached mindfulness.
- Conduct exposure exercises to survivors' worst fears.
- Address meta-cognitions such as positive and negative beliefs about worry.
- Encourage survivors to make plans for the future based on their values.

common therapeutic activities offered to manage high FCR are presented in Box 3.6.

There currently are very few interventions that have been developed and tested for care partners despite the documented prevalence of high FCR in this population. Preliminary research has demonstrated that care partners have different experiences with FCR than do patients[25] and that proper adaptations of patient interventions for use with care partners can be satisfactory and acceptable to these caregivers.[26]

Case Study

Paula is a 60-year-old woman who was diagnosed with stage 3 colon cancer after experiencing stomach cramps and noticing blood in her stools. Paula had surgery and chemotherapy and has been in follow-up for nearly 6 months, with no signs of recurrence. However, she often experiences stomach cramps that make her think her cancer has recurred and she palpates her abdomen daily to see if she can feel any lumps. Paula's worries get worse before attending follow-up appointments, but she doesn't want to bother her oncologist with her "silly" concerns. Paula completes psycho-social screening during her 6-month follow-up appointment, which includes the FCR-1r, and she scores 7/10, indicating possible clinical FCR. A nurse calls her after the appointment and notes that Paula seems quite worried about her cancer coming back, which she says is a common and understandable feeling for someone in her situation. She notes Paula's anxiety score was not particularly high and checks whether there is anything else Paula is worried about, which Paula denies. The nurse asks Paula how long she has been worried and whether she is still feeling worried since her appointment with the oncologist, in which her scans were clear. Paula says she feels a little less worried but mentions that she often thinks that her cancer has come back whenever she experiences symptoms and that she frequently checks her abdomen for lumps, which sometimes makes it hard for her to engage with home and work activities. The nurse sends Paula a link to complete the FCRI-SF online. Paula scores 25/36, indicating severe FCR. The nurse says that while it is normal to worry about cancer coming back, it seems like Paula's worries are quite severe and persistent and making her hypervigilant to physical symptoms. She asks whether Paula might be interested in talking to a psychologist. Paula agrees, and the nurse puts a referral into the hospital electronic medical record system, including the results of her assessments. She also adds a note to Paula's record for the oncologist to discuss symptom control with her at the next appointment. The nurse and Paula also discuss how Paula's constant checking for symptoms may actually be making her FCR worse, and they agree on a plan for the type, severity, and duration of symptoms that Paula needs to pay particular attention to and seek medical attention for.

Key Points from Case Study

- FCR is weakly linked to demographic and clinical characteristics, and patients may be reluctant to raise FCR, hence the need for proactive use of FCR screening tools.
- Physical symptoms are a common trigger for FCR, and hypervigilance to physical symptoms is a characteristic of clinical FCR.
- Health professionals should normalize FCR whenever possible.
- Heightened FCR around follow-up scans and appointments is common. If it persists beyond these times, it may be indicative of clinical FCR.
- Optimal care for FCR may involve management of both physical and psychological symptoms,
- Clear communication between the multidisciplinary team is important.

Professional Issues and Service Implementation

Recording and Communicating

- All assessments and treatments for FCR should be documented in accordance with the regulations of the healthcare provider delivering these services.
- Communication of FCR and the role of coping (e.g., seeking reassurance from healthcare professionals can provide temporary relief but increase FCR in the long run) to other professionals needs to follow duty-of-care requirements and keep the survivor's interests at the forefront.
- Discussion of recording of sessions, especially in the context of online/telehealth delivery, needs to be conducted at the inception of services.
- Because FCR can coexist with several psychiatric disorders, a thorough assessment is recommended. In some cases, more urgent clinical issues (e.g., suicidal urges, severe depression, unmanaged pain disorder) may need to be addressed first.
- While most clinicians surveyed during the development of criteria for clinical FCR did not support a psychiatric diagnosis of FCR,[10] in certain contexts (e.g., in the United States), a psychiatric diagnosis may be needed for FCR treatment to be reimbursed by insurers. In these cases, diagnosis

with an adjustment disorder, reflecting the understandable nature of fear after a major stressor (i.e., cancer diagnosis), may be considered.

Legal Responsibilities

Limits to confidentiality, especially in the context of virtual delivery of services, should be discussed before beginning services.

Common Ethical Dilemmas

FCR appears to differ across cultural groups.[27] There is a need for further validation and testing of FCR assessment tools and treatments in cultural and linguistic groups other than White English-speaking patients. While the list of tools and treatments being evaluated in culturally and linguistically diverse groups is growing (e.g., the FCRI is available in several languages), there is a dearth of research focused on addressing FCR in Indigenous peoples. Thus, clinicians need to be careful when applying assessment tools and interventions to survivors or caregivers belonging to groups other than White English-speaking populations.

Policies for Clinical Services

- A recently published FCR guideline outlines the considerable number of tools available for the identification, assessment, and management of FCR.[19] A complementary clinical pathway provides a step-by-step plan for the implementation of optimal care for FCR in clinical practice.[20] Embedding FCR screening tools in broader psychosocial screening programs is the first step in implementing care that is personalized for patients and efficient for healthcare professionals to deliver.

- FCR impacts care partners just as much and sometimes even more than it does patients.[28] Recognizing this need, assessing and addressing FCR in care partners is an emerging area of clinical practice and research. A caregiver-specific measure of FCR (the CARE-FCR)[29] has recently been validated, and some treatments are being adapted and pilot-tested with this population. However, centers will vary in their scope of practice in terms of available resources to address the needs of care partners. There are practical implementation issues to consider. Depending on availability of resources, healthcare teams may want to develop services within the hospital or cancer center for care partners or refer to existing community resources.

Teams and Supervision

🔍 Key Point

Cancer centers have many evidence-based options to choose from in terms of format and theoretical approaches to address clinical FCR: face-to-face, blended, individual, group, CBT, ACT, mindfulness based stress reduction (MBSR),[19] etc. Patient preference and the availability of existing resources may guide intervention selection in the absence of comparative trials assessing their differential efficacy.

🔍 Key Point

Training and supervising non–mental health specialists to triage patients and deliver care for mild to moderate FCR as part of a stepped-care model (i.e., a staged and tailored approach to delivering FCR care) will ensure that patients receive the optimal level of care for their FCR.[20]

References

1. https://canceratlas.cancer.org/the-burden/cancer-survivorship/?map= 7676. Accessed February 16, 2025.

2. Muzzin LJ, Anderson NJ, Figueredo AT, Gudelis SO. The experience of cancer. Soc Sci Med. 1994;38(9):1201–1208. doi: 10.1016/0277-9536(94)90185-6.

3. Lebel S, Ozakinci G, Humphris G, et al. From normal response to clinical problem: Definition and clinical features of fear of cancer recurrence. Support Care Cancer. 2016;24(8):3265–3268. doi: 10.1007/s00520-016-3272-5.

4. Coutts-Bain D, Sharpe L, Russell H. Death anxiety predicts fear of cancer recurrence and progression in ovarian cancer patients over and above other cognitive factors. J Behav Med. 2023;46(6):1023–1031. doi: 10.1007/s10865-023-00422-w.

5. Luigjes-Huizer YL, Tauber NM, Humphris G, et al. What is the prevalence of fear of cancer recurrence in cancer survivors and patients? A systematic review and individual participant data meta-analysis. Psycho-Oncol. 2022;31(6):879–892. doi: 10.1002/pon.5921.

6. Lee-Jones C, Humphris G, Dixon R, Hatcher MB. Fear of cancer recurrence: A literature review and proposed cognitive formulation to explain exacerbation of recurrence fears. Psycho-Oncol. 1997;6(2):95–105. doi: 10.1002/(SICI)1099-1611(199706)6:2<95::AID-PON250>3.0.CO;2-B.

7. Fardell JE, Thewes B, Turner J, et al. Fear of cancer recurrence: A theoretical review and novel cognitive processing formulation. J Cancer Surviv. 2016;10(4):663–673. doi: 10.1007/s11764-015-0512-5.

8. Curran, L., Sharpe, L., MacCann, C. et al. Testing a model of fear of cancer recurrence or progression: The central role of intrusions, death anxiety and threat appraisal. J Behav Med. 2020; 43: 225–236. doi: 10.1007/s10865-019-00129-x.

9. Simard S, Thewes B, Humphris G, et al. Fear of cancer recurrence in adult cancer survivors: A systematic review of quantitative studies. J Cancer Surviv. 2013;7(3):300–322. doi: 10.1007/s11764-013-0272-z.

10. Mutsaers B, Butow P, Dinkel A, et al. Identifying the key characteristics of clinical fear of cancer recurrence: An international Delphi study. Psycho-Oncol. 2020;29(2):430–436. doi: 10.1002/pon.5283.

11. American Psychiatric Association. Diagnostic and Statistical Manual of Mental Disorders (5th ed., text rev.). APA; 2022. https://doi.org/10.1176/appi.books.9780890425787

12. Rudy L, Maheu C, Körner A, Lebel S, Gélinas C. The FCR-1: Initial validation of a single-item measure of fear of cancer recurrence. Psycho-Oncol. 2020;29(4):788–795. doi: 10.1002/pon.5350.

13. Smith A', Gao M, Tran M, et al. Evaluation of the validity and screening performance of a revised single-item fear of cancer recurrence screening measure (FCR-1r). Psycho-Oncol. 2023;32(6):961–971. doi: 10.1002/pon.6139.

14. Simard S, Savard J. Screening and comorbidity of clinical levels of fear of cancer recurrence. J Cancer Surviv. 2015;9(3):481–491. doi: 10.1007/s11764-015-0424-4.

15. Humphris GM, Watson E, Sharpe M, Ozakinci G. Unidimensional scales for fears of cancer recurrence and their psychometric properties: The FCR4 and FCR7. Health Qual Life Outcomes. 2018;16(1):30. doi: 10.1186/s12955-018-0850-x.

16. Custers JAE, van den Berg SW, van Laarhoven HWM, Bleiker EMA, Gielissen MFM, Prins JB. The Cancer Worry Scale: Detecting fear of recurrence in breast cancer survivors. Cancer Nurs. 2014;37(1):E44–E50. doi: 10.1097/NCC.0b013e3182813a17.

17. Simard S, Savard J. Screening and comorbidity of clinical levels of fear of cancer recurrence. J Cancer Surviv. 2015;9(3):481–491. doi: 10.1007/s11764-015-0424-4.

18. Giguère L, Mutsaers B, Harris C, et al. The Ottawa clinical fear of recurrence instruments: A screener, self-report, and clinical interview. Psycho-Oncol. 2024;33(6):e6364. doi: 10.1002/pon.6364.

19. Lebel S, Zwaal C, Craig L, Conrod R, Freeman J, Galica C, Maheu C, Nissin R, Savard J. Fear of Cancer Recurrence guideline. Cancer Care Ontario. 2024. https://www.cancercareontario.ca/en/guidelines-advice/types-of-cancer/75576

20. Smith A, Girgis A, Taylor N, et al. Step-by-step: A clinical pathway for stepped care management of fear of cancer recurrence-results of a three-round online delphi consensus process with Australian health professionals and researchers. J Cancer Surviv. Published online October 7, 2024. doi: 10.1007/s11764-024-01685-1.

21. Liu JJ, Butow P, Beith J. Systematic review of interventions by non-mental health specialists for managing fear of cancer recurrence in adult cancer survivors. Support Care Cancer. 2019;27(11):4055–4067. doi: 10.1007/s00520-019-04979-8.

22. Butow PN, Turner J, Gilchrist J, et al. Randomized trial of ConquerFear: A novel, theoretically based psychosocial intervention for fear of cancer recurrence. J Clin Oncol. 2017;35(36):4066–4077. doi: 10.1200/JCO.2017.73.1257.

23. Tauber NM, O'Toole MS, Dinkel A, et al. Effect of psychological intervention on fear of cancer recurrence: A systematic review and meta-analysis. J Clin Oncol. 2019;37(31):2899–2915. doi: 10.1200/JCO.19.00572.

24. Hall DL, Luberto CM, Philpotts LL, Song R, Park ER, Yeh GY. Mind-body interventions for fear of cancer recurrence: A systematic review and meta-analysis. Psycho-Oncol. 2018;27(11):2546–2558. doi: 10.1002/pon.4757.

25. Webb K, Sharpe L, Butow P, et al. Caregiver fear of cancer recurrence: A systematic review and meta-analysis of quantitative studies. Psycho-Oncol. 2023;32(8):1173–1191. doi: 10.1002/pon.6176.

26. Lamarche J, Nissim R, Avery J, et al. It is time to address fear of cancer recurrence in family caregivers: Feasibility and acceptability of a randomized pilot study of the family caregiver version of the Fear of Recurrence Therapy (FC-FORT). Psycho-Oncol. 2025;34(2):e70084. doi: 10.1002/pon.70084.

27. Anderson K, Smith A, Diaz A, et al. A systematic review of fear of cancer recurrence among Indigenous and minority peoples. Front Psychol. 2021;12:621850. doi: 10.3389/fpsyg.2021.621850.

28. Smith A, Wu VS, Lambert S, et al. A systematic mixed studies review of fear of cancer recurrence in families and caregivers of adults diagnosed with cancer. J Cancer Surviv. 2022;16(6):1184–1219. doi: 10.1007/s11764-021-01109-4.

29. Webb K, Sharpe L, Russell H, Shaw J. Development and validation of the CARE-FCR: A caregiver-specific measure of fear of cancer recurrence and progression. Psycho-Oncol. 2024;33(4):e6341. doi: 10.1002/pon.6341.

Further Reading and Resources

1. Bergerot C, et al. Fear of cancer recurrence or progression: What is it and what can we do about it? Am Soc Clin Oncol Educ Book. 2022;42:18–27. doi: 10.1200/EDBK_100031.

   A comprehensive review of FCR theories, assessment tools and interventions.

2. Butow P, et al. Fear of cancer recurrence: A practical guide for clinicians. Oncol J. 2018;32(1):32–38.

   Useful suggestions of how oncology clinicians can address FCR in routine encounters.

3. Mutsaers B, et al. Assessing and managing patient fear of cancer recurrence. Can Fam Physician. 2020;66(9):672–673.

   A resource to help primary care physicians address FCR with cancer patients.

4. FORT: Psychosocial Oncology Laboratory. To request materials from the Fear of Cancer Recurrence Therapy (FORT), including patient and facilitator manuals and training videos. https://www.psolab.ca/fort

5. Fear of Cancer Recurrence Hub: PoCoG. To request material from the Conquer Fear intervention, including manuals and handouts. https://www.pocog.org.au/fear-of-cancer-recurrence-hub

Chapter 4

Depressive Disorders

Daisuke Fujisawa and Tatsuo Akechi

Learning Objectives

After reading this chapter, the clinician will be able to

1. Understand the signs and symptoms of depression in cancer survivors.
2. Conduct a comprehensive assessment of depressive disorders and consider differential diagnoses.
3. Understand basic principles of psychotherapy and pharmacotherapy for depression in patients with cancer.
4. Describe ethical, cultural, legal, and professional issues linked to clinical care of patients with depression in the cancer survivorship context.

Background Evidence

Depression is a common syndrome among patients with cancer with reported prevalence being between 5% and 60%.[1] The prevalence of major depression (major depressive disorder) according to stringent criteria is 16.3% (13.419.5%), with another 19.2% (9.1–31.9%) suffering from minor depression (a milder type of depression or adjustment disorder).[2] These figures are two to three times higher than the general population and are similar to those in patients with other physical illness.[3]

Depression impairs patients' well-being in many ways. Even a mild level of depression can cause significant decrements in quality of life comparable to those due to physical symptoms and decreased performance status.[4] Depression is associated with poorer health outcomes and shorter survival in cancer patients due to both death by cancer and by other causes.[5] Lower survival of patients with depression is partly explained by poorer adherence to cancer treatment and recommended follow-up and unfavorable lifestyle, such as decreased levels of physical exercise, higher alcohol consumption, or inappropriate diet, which may lead to higher physical comorbidities. Depression often increases sensitivity to and monitoring of physical sensations and thereby may increase pain perception. Depression is a large contributor to suicide.

Both biological and psychosocial factors are involved in depression.[6] Recent evidence indicates that inflammatory cytokines contribute to the development of depression. Increased levels of inflammation and pro-inflammatory cytokines (such as C-reactive protein [CRP], tumor necrosis factor [TNF-alpha], interleukin-6 [IL-6], and IL-1beta) caused by cancer can lead to alterations in neurotransmitters such as the monoamine, glutamate, neuropeptide systems, and brain-derived growth factor (BDNF).

Psychosocial challenges that cancer survivors face, such as symptom burden and functional decline due to residual symptoms, long-term adverse effects, changed body image, and difficulty in social reintegration, may lead to the development of depression.

Depression, especially severe depression, is frequently underrecognized and undertreated since patients with depression tend to express their emotions less than those without depression. Therefore, routine screening is considered vital in oncology practice.[7]

Evidence provides modest support for pharmacotherapy (mainly antidepressants) in the treatment of depression in cancer settings.[8] Psychotherapy has a stronger evidence base than pharmacotherapy and thus is considered first-line treatment when it is available.[9,10] Mindfulness-based psychotherapies and a range of complementary therapies are also employed.[11] Technology-based and online therapies are beginning to make their contributions.[12]

Presenting Problems

Key Symptoms and Signs

Depression is a syndrome characterized by depressed mood and anhedonia (decreased interest or diminished sense of pleasure). It is a spectrum of symptoms in which normal sadness or grief occurs at the milder end and major depressive disorder at the opposite, more severe end. Minor or subthreshold depression lies in the middle. The diagnostic criteria for major depressive disorder are shown in Box 4.1.

A patient is diagnosed with minor (or subthreshold) depression when two to four of these symptoms are present for at least 2 weeks. A state whereby three to four depressive symptoms are present continuously for at least 2 years is called *dysthymia* (chronic depression). The diagnostic term "adjustment disorder" is often used for milder forms of depression. It refers to a state of moderate to marked distress that is greater than expected from exposure to a stressor and may present with depressive symptoms (see Chapter 2 for details of adjustment disorders). Though life stressors may provide "good reasons" for sadness—such as being diagnosed with cancer—the diagnosis of depression should be made if a patient meets the criteria for major or minor depression.

Supporting symptoms of depressive disorders (and not nonpathological emotional reactions to stressful events) include more pervasive symptoms of depression, loss of emotional reactivity to good news, irrational sense of self-guilt (e.g., patients who believe it is their fault that they have cancer), and

Box 4.1 Symptomatology of Major Depressive Disorder

1. Depressed mood
2. Anhedonia (lack of interest or pleasure in almost all activities)
3. Sleep disorder (insomnia or hypersomnia)
4. Appetite loss, weight loss, or, conversely, appetite gain, weight gain
5. Fatigue or loss of energy
6. Psychomotor retardation (patient looks slow in actions or responses) or agitation (patient looks irritable and hasty)
7. Trouble concentrating or trouble making decisions
8. Low self-esteem or feelings of guilt
9. Recurrent thoughts of death or suicidal ideation

Five symptoms from the above list are required to make the diagnosis of depression and must include depressed mood and/or anhedonia

Note: The symptoms must have been present most of the day, nearly every day, for at least 2 weeks. The symptoms cannot be explained by other physical or psychiatric problems.

Source: Abstracted from *Diagnostic and Statistical Manual of Mental Disorders*, Fifth Edition, Text Revision (DSM-5-TR), American Psychiatric Association; 2022.

persistent suicidal thoughts, possibly with concrete plans. Depressed patients often have physical symptoms (so-called neurovegetative symptoms), such as sleep disturbance, psychomotor retardation, appetite disturbance, poor concentration, and low energy.

Making a Formal Diagnosis

The diagnosis of depression must be made by clinical interviews according to the criteria of either the *Diagnostic and Statistical Manual of Mental Disorders* (DSM-5-TR) or the *International Classification of Diseases* (ICD-11). Formally, clinicians may refer to a manual of the Structured Clinical Interview for the DSM-5-TR, while in actual clinical practice clinicians usually simply ask whether a patient has each symptom of depression, as listed by the DSM-5-TR or ICD-11. *Clinicians start by asking about the core symptoms of depression (depressive mood and anhedonia). The presence of either of these two symptoms ought to prompt clinicians to perform a full diagnostic assessment for major depression.*

Issues Surrounding Diagnosing Depression in Cancer Patients

Many symptoms of depression, such as loss of appetite, loss of weight, and loss of energy, overlap with symptoms caused by cancer or cancer treatment. The rule of thumb is to diagnose a patient as depressed and offer a therapeutic trial of treatment unless there is clear evidence that a person's depressive symptoms come from physical issues, thus avoiding the chance of failing to treat (inclusive approach). There have, however, been continuing debates regarding the need to modify the DSM criteria of major depression when applied to cancer survivors.[13]

Screening Tools for Depression

Screening for depression can be done by clinician assessment or self-administered questionnaires. Shorter screening tools (ultra-short screeners) are easy to administer, but their specificity in diagnosing depression tends to be low; thus they should be followed by further clinical assessments. Longer screening tools tend to perform better in specificity than shorter screening tools, but they cannot substitute for formal clinical interviews.

The instruments widely used in oncology settings include but are not limited to the following[14]:

* *Two-question methods (ultra-short):* The US Preventive Services Task Force recommends the following two-item screening for major depression:
  "Over the past 2 weeks, have you ever felt down, depressed, or hopeless?"
  "Over the past 2 weeks, have you felt little interest or pleasure doing things?
* *Distress Thermometer (DT) (ultra-short):* The DT is an 11-point numeric scale that mimics a thermometer on which the patients self-rate their distress. The National Comprehensive Cancer Network (NCCN) guidelines recommend a distress score of 4 out of 10 as a cutoff. Some modified versions of the DT, such as the Distress and Impact Thermometer (DIT), are also used as a screening tool in some countries.
* *Patient Health Questionnaire (PHQ-9 and PHQ-2):* The PHQ-9 is a screening questionnaire comprising nine questions that correspond to symptoms of DSM-5 major depression. A score of 10 or higher has demonstrated 88% sensitivity and 88% specificity for the diagnosis of major depression. The PHQ-2 is a two-item, ultra-short questionnaire that extracts two core symptoms of depression (depressed mood and anhedonia) from the PHQ-9.
* *Hospital Anxiety and Depression Scale (HADS):* The HADS is a 14-item self-rating questionnaire that asks about symptoms of depression and anxiety. It is the most widely used measure for depression in oncology settings. It does not include somatic symptoms, thus eliminating the influence of physical conditions. The threshold to define depression is a subscale score of 11 or above (8–10 is "borderline").
* *Beck Depression Inventory (BDI):* The BDI is often considered the "gold standard" scale for depression. Its limitations include its length (21 items), which can reduce acceptability, and the inclusion of somatic symptoms, which can reduce specificity. The BDI-Short Form (BDI-SF), a shorter form of BDI, with the number of physical symptom items reduced, has benefits in oncology practice. Scores of 0–3 on BDI-SF indicate minimal depression; 4–6 indicate mild depression; 7–9 indicate moderate depression; and 10–21 indicate severe depression.[15]

Key Problems Associated with Development of Depression

Depression can occur in patients with any type of cancer and at any stage of illness. Key risk factors for depression include

* past history of depression or other psychiatric disorders
* family history of depression
* higher symptom burden (e.g., late and persisting adverse effects of treatment)

- more frequent unmet needs (e.g., physical, social, psychological, and spiritual)
- lower socioeconomic status

Investigations for Key Differential Diagnoses

Key Differentials
Key differentials for depression are shown in Box 4.2.

Essential Tests
The essential tests for the differential diagnoses of depression are shown in Box 4.3. However, clinicians should judiciously select examination items according to the patients' physical condition and available treatments.

Further Assessments
Depressed patients, especially older patients and those with severe depressive symptoms, may not explicitly admit to lowered mood, which can make the assessment difficult.

🔍 Key Point
The following objective appearance and behaviors in patients may be signs of depression.
- Social withdrawal
- Not participating in medical care
- Diminished positive emotional reactions (e.g., not able to be cheered up; does not smile; no response to good news, visitors, or funny situations)
- Demeanor shows reduced facial reactivity and slowed thinking
- Wish for hastened death

Factors that Contribute to Misdiagnosis or Inappropriate Care: Fatigue and Devastating Physical Conditions
Fatigue is one of the most common symptoms in cancer survivors and it mimics depression. See Table 4.1 for tips to differentiate depression from fatigue. In cases of uncertainty, an empiric trial of antidepressant therapy may be worthwhile to ensure that a patient with possible depression is not left untreated.

Clinical Management

Screening and Referral
The clinical approach to depression begins with routine screening followed by detailed assessment and appropriate treatment according to the severity of depression. Routine screening should be administered at critical time points during cancer care (e.g., after receiving bad news, during transition from one

Box 4.2 Key Differential Diagnoses for Depression

Physical Conditions
- Unresolved physical distress (e.g., pain, nausea)
- Endocrine dysfunction (e.g., hyperthyroidism, hypothyroidism, adrenal insufficiency), which can be caused by either surgical resection, radiation therapy, immune therapies, or cancer metastases.
- Anemia
- Diabetes mellitus
- Nutritional deficiency (vitamin B_3 [nicotinic acid, niacin], vitamin B_{12}, folate, vitamin C)
- Electrolyte imbalance (sodium, potassium, calcium, magnesium)
- Certain cancers causing cytokine cascades (C-reactive protein [CRP], low albumin)
- Cancer-related fatigue
- Other exhausting physical conditions, such as cardiac dysfunction, hepatic dysfunction, infection, pulmonary dysfunction

Organic Brain Disorders
- Cancer-related:
  - Brain tumor or metastasis, especially frontal lobe apathy
  - Meningitis carcinomatosis or leptomeningeal disease
  - Paraneoplastic syndromes
- Other neurological disorders:
  - Parkinson's syndrome, multiple sclerosis, HIV encephalopathy, cerebrovascular diseases, etc.
- Changed mental status:
  - Consciousness disturbance, including delirium (especially hypoactive delirium)

Other Psychiatric/Psychological States
- Alcohol/substance abuse (chronic alcohol abuse can cause depressive symptoms, which can be alleviated by abstinence)
- Normal grief (normal psychological reaction to stress)
- Demoralization syndrome (see Chapter 2)

Medication Side Effects
- Steroids, interferon, beta-adrenergic blockers, calcium-channel blockers, barbiturates, cholinergic medications, estrogens
- Late effect of anticancer agents ("chemobrain")

Medication Withdrawal
- Steroids
- Stimulants

Box 4.3 Essential Tests for Diagnosing Major Depression

- Laboratory tests to exclude:
  - Anemia (Hb, Ht)
  - Electrolyte disturbance (Na, K, Ca, Mg)
  - Hypoglycemia (Glu)
  - Endocrine disorders (thyroid tests [TSH, fT3, fT4], ACTH, cortisol)
  - Liver and renal dysfunction (AST, ALT, BUN, Cr)
  - Acute and chronic inflammation (CRP)
  - Malnutrition and absorption disturbance (vitamin B_1, B_{12}, folate)
  - Malnutrition and frailty (albumin)
- Neuroimaging: Computed tomography (CT) brain scan, magnetic resonance imaging (MRI) brain scan (Gd-enhancement is recommended to detect subtle brain metastasis, leptomeningeal disease, or meningitis carcinomatosis)
- Electroencephalogram: When consciousness disturbance or epilepsy (psychomotor seizure) is suspected
- Other imaging studies and/or biomarkers to exclude cancer recurrence when appropriate

Table 4.1 Distinguishing fatigue from depression

Clinical state	Key features
Fatigue	
	Patients are usually able to derive some pleasure from activities with low physical burden and from activities that they normally found enjoyable.
	More motivated when physical symptoms are mild.
	Late afternoon is the most difficult time of the day.
	Higher prevalence than depression.
Depression	
	Patients are unable to experience pleasure from experiences that they used to enjoy.
	Morning is the most difficult time of the day.
	Persistent suicidal thoughts, pervasive feeling of guilt and hopelessness may be seen.
	Prior history and family history of depression increase the likelihood of developing an episode of depression.

Caveat: fatigue and depression may be concurrent.

treatment modality to another). Following such screening, comprehensive assessment and support should be provided.

Comprehensive Assessment and Coordination of Care

Good communication between clinicians and patients is fundamental to preventing and alleviating depression. Proactive, comprehensive assessments should be made to cover multiple domains of patients' needs and concerns. Intervention can be delivered in different forms, including basic support, education, problem-solving, counseling, and specialist consultations. Working in multidisciplinary teams consisting of physicians, nurses, social workers, nutritionists, rehabilitation therapists, counselors, and psycho-oncologists is mandatory for proper psychosocial cancer care.

Treatment

The two major treatment modalities of depression are psychotherapy and pharmacotherapy. Their indications are considered based on severity of depression, physical conditions, patient preference, and access to care. Psychotherapy (psychological treatment) is indicated at all levels of depression severity. It is usually preferred in milder cases since it requires patients' active participation and it may take a longer time than psychotropic medication to be effective. Psychotherapy outperforms pharmacotherapy in relapse-prevention effect, which means that the effect of psychotherapy is sustained even after the treatment ends. Pharmacotherapy usually takes a shorter time than psychotherapy to come to effect, and its effect size is larger in more severe cases. Therefore, pharmacotherapy is considered an essential treatment for severe depression and an optional treatment for mild to moderate depression. A patient's physical conditions, such as comorbidities and vulnerabilities, may limit the use of pharmacotherapy.

Psychotherapy

General Principles

Before implementing a psychotherapeutic strategy, it is important to develop a formulation and to consider whether the patient is eligible for psychotherapy, what type of psychotherapy is most suitable, and what the patient's preferences for the treatment approach are. Generally, patients need to be motivated enough to commit to the therapy, and the symptoms of depression should not hinder their ability to take part in the therapy (e.g., a patient is not too fatigued to talk). A fuller explanation of different therapies can be found in the *Handbook of Psychotherapy in Cancer Care* (see Further Reading).

Cognitive Behavioral Therapy

Cognitive behavioral therapy (CBT), or cognitive therapy, is a structured psychotherapy based on the hypothesis that one's emotional and somatic responses (mood and physical symptoms) are determined by how one perceives a situation (cognition) rather than the situation itself. CBT involves practicing relaxation techniques, enhancing problem-solving skills, and identifying and correcting unhelpful or dysfunctional thoughts and behaviors associated with negative feelings and distressing physical symptoms. There is robust evidence that CBT is effective for patients with cancer.[16]

Behavioral activation (BA), as part of CBT, also decreases depression in patients with cancer.[17] The rationale of BA is that people who are depressed struggle with loss of energy, motivation, and opportunities for feeling pleasure or a sense of achievement. The therapist encourages patients to undertake activities that bring them pleasure or feelings of achievement by encouraging them to develop a schedule of daily activities and monitor mood changes that result from each activity.

Problem-Solving Therapy

Problem-solving therapy (PST) is often described as a simpler or more focused form of CBT and is based on the hypothesis that psychological distress is linked with unsolved problems; therefore, acquisition of efficient problem-solving (or coping) strategies leads to decreased distress. The therapist teaches methods of efficacious problem-solving, which is achieved through

1. Defining the problem,
2. Brainstorming possible options,
3. Evaluating potential solutions by weighing the advantages and disadvantages of each solution,
4. Implementing specific solutions,
5. Evaluating their degree of success, and
6. Fine-tuning them.

Since this is a quite straightforward method, it can be implemented by health professionals who are not specialized in mental health (e.g., primary care nurses) and who have completed relatively short training.[18]

Mindfulness-Based Therapies

Mindfulness-based interventions (MBIs) are increasingly being integrated into oncological treatment to mitigate psychological distress and promote emotional and physical well-being. Common protocols used are mindfulness-based stress reduction (MBSR), mindfulness-based cognitive therapy (MBCT), and mindfulness-based cancer recovery (MBCR) treatments.[11]

Other Psychotherapies

A variety of psychotherapies have been applied to patients with cancer. Some examples of psychotherapies with a stronger evidence-base, in both general and oncology practice, include supportive psychotherapy, interpersonal psychotherapy (IPT), acceptance and commitment therapy (ACT), and family and couples therapy (see Chapter 6 for a description of different psychotherapies).

Pharmacotherapy

General Principles

Antidepressants are the first choice of drugs for adult depression. This also applies to depressed patients who have comorbid cancer, although further clinical trials in this population are needed to draw firm conclusions.[9,10] Antidepressants must be taken daily and require 4–6 weeks to achieve full effect. Treatment failure should not be declared before a minimum of 4–6 weeks of treatment once the maximum dose is administered. The most common reason for poor response is inadequate upward titration of the dosage.

The medication should be continued for at least 6 months after reaching recovery to prevent the relapse of depression. Antidepressants should be reduced gradually since discontinuation syndrome can occur within days after rapidly stopping selective serotonin reuptake inhibitors (SSRIs), serotonin norepinephrine reuptake inhibitors (SNRIs), and tricyclic antidepressants (TCAs). Typical symptoms of discontinuation syndrome are "flu-like symptoms" (e.g., dizziness, nausea, fatigue, muscle aches, chills), anxiety and irritability, sleep disturbance, and cardiac arrythmia. Readministration of the drug alleviates those symptoms.

Rotating medications or supplementing with adjunctive medications may be indicated if there has not been enough response by 6–12 weeks at maximal dose. Examples of augmentation therapies for antidepressants include lithium, lamotrigine, buspirone, psychostimulants, and low-dose neuroleptics.

Antidepressants

Choice of an Agent

There are a few categories ("class") of antidepressants. No single antidepressant is universally accepted as more effective than another despite some variation in their effectiveness and acceptability. Many antidepressants are metabolized by CYP 450 enzymes; thus, clinicians should be watchful for potential interactions with other medications in use (see Table 4.2).

🔍 Key Point

Initial choice of an agent should be based on adverse effects, interactions with other medications, dosing schedule, and history of effective response.

Usually, SSRIs, SNRIs, or mirtazapine are used as first-choice drugs. Treatment adherence and treatment response should be monitored frequently (e.g., twice a month or more) especially at the beginning of treatment and in severely depressed or suicidal patients.

Dosage and Treatment Plan

Start at a low dose and titrate upward gradually, especially for elderly or vulnerable patients, usually at a pace of 1–2 weeks (see Table 4.3). SSRIs and SNRIs frequently cause nausea or emesis at the beginning of administration. Clinicians should inform patients that nausea or emesis may occur but usually resolves within a few days.

- *SSRIs/SNRIs*: SSRIs are the most frequently prescribed antidepressants. Postcibal administration (e.g., taken after breakfast) reduces the risk of nausea. Antiemetic drugs (e.g., mosapride, metoclopramide) can be prescribed for these side effects. Other common adverse effects include sleep disturbance (either insomnia or hypersomnia) and sexual dysfunction. Since serotonin associates with platelet aggregation, administration of SSRIs can increase the risk of bleeding, especially in patients who are already taking nonsteroidal anti-inflammatory drugs (NSAIDs) or other antiplatelet medications. The syndrome of inappropriate antidiuretic hormone secretion (SIADH) can be caused by SSRIs, SNRIs, and TCAs and presents with a low sodium level.

  In a small group of individuals, SSRIs and SNRIs may cause irritability, agitation, or dysphoria at the beginning of administration ("activation syndrome"). This can be alleviated by decreasing the dose, switching medicine,

Table 4.2 Types of antidepressants and their characteristics

Drug type	Actions	Therapeutics	Side effects, contraindications	Agents
Serotonin reuptake inhibitors (SSRIs)	Blocks reuptake of serotonin (5HT) at serotonin transporter	Common initial treatment of depression. Generally mild adverse effects. Also effective for anxiety disorders	Nausea/emesis and sexual dysfunction are common. May lead to weigh gain, agitation, platelet dysfunction, insomnia or sedation.	Citalopram, escitalopram, fluoxetine, fluvoxamine, paroxetine, sertraline
Serotonin norepinephrine reuptake inhibitors (SNRIs)	Blocks reuptake of 5HT and norepinephrine (NE) at 5HT and NE transporters	Generally mild adverse effects. Also effective for neuropathic pain	High blood pressure at higher doses	Desvenlafaxine, venlafaxine, duloxetine
Mirtazapine	Agonist at alpha-2 adrenergic and 5HT-2a, -2c, -3 auto receptors to facilitate release of NE and 5HT, Blocks histamine (H_1) receptors	Useful for patients with anorexia and/or insomnia	May cause weight gain, sedation, autonomic effects	Mirtazapine
Bupropion	Blocks uptake of dopamine (DA) and NE	Useful as an adjunct to SSRIs. Helps with smoking cessation.	Lowered seizure threshold at higher doses (therefore limited in palliative care)	Bupropion
TCAs	Blocks reuptake of 5HT and NE	Secondary option for otherwise resistant depression. Limited use today, except as a co-analgesic.	Anticholinergic effects (constipation, urinary retention, confusion), arrythmia and weight gain. (contraindicated for glaucoma, past myocardial infarction, and diabetes)	Amitriptyline, clomipramine, desipramine, dothiepin, doxepin, imipramine, nortriptyline, protriptyline, trimipramine
Monoamine oxidase inhibitors (MAOIs)	Prolonged anti-MAO-A/B actions	Third-line treatment for resistant depression; not used in palliative care	Autonomic and sexual effects, anticholinergic effects	Phenelzine, tranylcypromine

Table 4.3 Initial and regular dose of medications

Medication	Initial dose (mg/day)	Dosing range (mg/day)	Key drug interactions
Selective serotonin reuptake inhibitors (SSRIs)			**Caution with NSAIDS (risk of bleeding) and diuretics (SIADH)**
Citalopram	10–20	20–60	
Escitalopram	5–10	10–20	
Fluoxetine	10–20	20–80	CYP 2D6 inhibition (may affect tamoxifen and abiraterone metabolism)
Fluvoxamine	25–50	50–300	
Paroxetine	10–20	20–60 (CR: 2.5–62.5)	CYP 2D6 inhibition (may affect tamoxifen and abiraterone metabolism)
Sertraline	25–50	50–200	CYP 2D6 inhibition (may affect tamoxifen and abiraterone metabolism)
Serotonin norepinephrine reuptake inhibitors (SNRIs)			**Caution with ciprofloxacin, ketoconazole**
Desvenlafaxine	50	50–200	
Duloxetine	20	40–120	
Venlafaxine	75	25–300	
Other antidepressants			
Bupropion	25–50	150–450	May lower seizure threshold
Buspirone	15	15–60	
Mirtazapine	15	15–45	
Psychostimulants			**Caution with antihypertensive medications, clonidine, anticoagulants, steroids, anticonvulsants**
Methylphenidate	5–10 am	20 am	
Modafinil	50–100 am	100–200 am	

or concurrently prescribing benzodiazepines. SSRIs, SNRIs, and TCAs should be discontinued gradually to prevent discontinuation syndrome.

• *Mirtazapine*: In contrast to SSRIs and SNRIs, mirtazapine does not cause nausea or emesis. Rather, it increases appetite and is favored by patients who suffer from appetite loss. Sleepiness is another common adverse effect that can be either harmful or helpful for patients depending on their situation (i.e., somnolence can decrease a patient's function but can be helpful for those who suffer from insomnia).

- *Bupropion*: Bupropion is often used as an adjunct to SSRIs. It also helps with smoking cessation.
- *Tricyclics*: TCAs are older-generation antidepressants that have more frequent adverse effects and lower tolerability. Since their effectiveness is not significantly different from those of newer-generation antidepressants, TCAs are seldom used as a first-line antidepressant.
- *Monoamine oxidase inhibitors*: MAO-Is have many harmful adverse effects (autonomic effects and dietary restrictions [avoid tyramine]) and are thus considered a third-line treatment for treatment-resistant depression.
- *Benzodiazepines*: Benzodiazepines are commonly used anxiolytics, and they may be used as an adjunct to antidepressants to alleviate distress, anxiety, and/or agitation. Their quick effect is considered favorable by patients and clinicians, although effectiveness for depression in the long term (>4 weeks) has not been proved. Benzodiazepines are also frequently used as hypnotics.

  Common adverse effects of benzodiazepines are sleepiness, fatigue, and decreased concentration, which can impair daily functioning. They may also cause dizziness and muscle weakness, leading to an elevated risk of falls. Benzodiazepines may induce delirium in vulnerable patients and patients with cognitive decline.
- *Buspirone*: Buspirone is another anxiolytic whose adverse effects are milder than benzodiazepines. Its effectiveness as a sole agent in treating depression is limited, but it can be used adjunctively with SSRIs.
- *Neuroleptics*: Neuroleptics (antipsychotics) are used either as augmentation therapy for depression or as an alternative for anxiolytics, especially in patients with severe symptoms that cannot be alleviated by benzodiazepines or in patients at risk of dependence using benzodiazepines. Some neuroleptics (e.g., quetiapine, aripiprazole) themselves have antidepressant effects. Their potential adverse effects include extrapyramidal symptoms (Parkinsonian syndrome) and weight gain.
- *Psychostimulants*: Psychostimulants such as methylphenidate and modafinil may be used alone if rapid onset is needed, in combination with antidepressants to achieve rapid initial response, or as an adjunct. They are also used to counter the fatigue or sedation caused by opioids.[11]
- *Other agents*: The following agents may be indicated in specific situations, such as when a patient needs immediate resolution of depression (e.g., a patient is seriously suicidal) or when a series of antidepressants are ineffective or contraindicated.
  - *Ketamine*: Administered intravenously, subcutaneously, or intranasally. Indicated for depressed patients who are resistant to antidepressants or who need immediate resolution of depression. Ketamine may also be effective for pain management.[9]
  - *Cannabis*: Cannabis may be prescribed in some jurisdictions, although so far there is no supportive evidence base to prescribe cannabis for the treatment of depression.

- *Psilocybin*: Psychedelic-assisted therapy using psilocybin can be used in treating anxiety, depression, and existential distress in patients with life-threatening illness.[10] Psychedelic drugs are currently illegal in many countries and are awaiting further research for their clinical indications.

Electroconvulsive Therapy and other Neuromodulation Therapies

Electroconvulsive therapy (ECT) induces a controlled seizure through the use of electrical stimulation to the brain while the patient is under anesthesia. It is a treatment of choice for patients with depression refractory to pharmacotherapy, patients with psychotic depression, patients who are acutely suicidal, and vulnerable patients who cannot tolerate standard pharmacotherapy.

Other neuromodulation therapies for depression include transcranial magnetic stimulation (TMS) and transcranial direct current stimulation (tDCS). TMS stimulates the prefrontal cortex through an induced magnetic field. The treatment is usually given approximately 5 days a week for 4–6 weeks. tDCS induces a weak constant-current electric flow through the cerebral cortex via scalp electrodes; the current modulates cortical excitability and spontaneous neural activity. Although clinical evidence of these therapies in oncology settings has been scarce, they may be applicable in some situations and when available.

Complementary and Integrative Therapies

MBIs, yoga, music therapy, relaxation, and reflexology are recommended for patients undergoing cancer treatment, and MBIs, yoga, and tai chi and/or qi-gong are recommended post-treatment, although the methodological quality of the referenced studies is generally low except for MBIs.[19, 22]

Case Study

A 70-year-old man who underwent resection surgery for esophageal cancer 2 months earlier was referred to a psycho-oncologist because he persistently complained of dysphagea—sense of choking and that "the food gets stuck in the chest and does not go down"—even though there were no remarkable findings to support his complaints on esophageal endoscopy and video-fluoroscopic examination of swallowing. His family was concerned that he had been extremely inactive, and he looked agonized all day. He lost more than 10 Kg in weight. He said he would be better off dead if this agony continued. A close interview revealed a persistent depressive mood, lack of appetite, poor sleep, and a sense of guilt that "life is not worth living."

The patient was diagnosed as having major depression, and mirtazapine 7.5 mg (before sleep) was started. His sleep and appetite began to improve after a few days. Although the patient's mood improved a bit and his physical complaints diminished after a few weeks, he was hesitant to get out of bed because he felt "too fatigued to move." Mirtazapine was switched to duloxetine since an adverse effect (drowsiness and fatigue) was suspected. In collaboration with the rehabilitation team, the patient was encouraged to gradually increase his activity level based on the principles of behavioral activation (see later sections for detail).

The patient, his family, and nurses created an activity schedule that initially included small activities and later increased. Detailed conversations with the patient revealed that his unwillingness to get up arose from a sense of dizziness and fear of falling, probably caused by inactivity leading to weakened muscle strength. Following assessment by the interdisciplinary team and reassurance from his treating physician, the patient became more active after a week and started participating in rehabilitation.

Professional Issues and Service Implementation

Impact of Depression on Mental Capacity

Depression, especially severe depression, interferes with patients' cognition and may impair their decision-making capacity. Clinicians should be watchful whether a patient's decisions and behavior are negatively influenced by depression.

Suicide and Wish for Hastened Death

Depression is a contributor to the wish for hastened death (e.g., through suicide, physician-assisted suicide, euthanasia, or rejection of proper treatment). It is not always easy to discriminate clinical depression from a patient's natural response to tough physical conditions. Prioritize the diagnosis of depression in order not to miss the chance of recovery that can be attained.

🔍 Key Point

If a patient is suspected of being at heightened risk of suicide, clinicians are responsible for referring such patients to an appropriate mental healthcare specialist. Intensive psychiatric care, including admission to a psychiatric ward, may be indicated. Involving the caregivers of such patients in care coordination is required.

Teams and Supervision

Regardless of whether the patient is diagnosed as depressed, any bio- or psychosocial problems and concerns should be addressed using an interdisciplinary approach. Detection and management of depression may be best done by collaboration between front-line medical providers (e.g., primary care physicians or oncologists) and a trained "care manager" (e.g., trained nurses) who works under the supervision of consultant psychiatrists. A typical program of this "collaborative care model"[20, 23] starts with the administration of a self-report screening questionnaire for depression to all the patients in a clinic. If a patient reports high emotional distress, they receive a face-to-face or telephone diagnostic interview for depression by trained staff. If the patient is diagnosed with depression, they are provided with psychoeducation for depression and brief psychotherapy (e.g., problem-solving therapy) in addition to practical advice on managing life with cancer and psychological distress. When clinically relevant, a report is generated for the patient's primary care provider. Also, guidance about the use of psychotropics is provided by the care managers under the supervision of psychiatrists.

References

1. Caruso R, Nanni MG, Riba M, et al. Depressive spectrum disorders in cancer: Prevalence, risk factors and screening for depression: a critical review. Acta Oncol 2017;56(2):146–155.

2. Mitchell AJ, Chan M, Bhatti H, et al. Prevalence of depression, anxiety, and adjustment disorder in oncological, haematological, and palliative-care settings: A meta-analysis of 94 interview-based studies. Lancet Oncol. 2011;12(2):160–174.

3. National Institute for Health and Care Excellence (NICE): Depression in adults with a chronic physical health problem: recognition and management (CG91), NICE 2009. Clinical guideline. October 28, 2009. nice.org.uk/guidance/cg91

4. Fujisawa D, Inoguchi H, Shimoda H, et al. Impact of depression on health utility value in cancer patients. Psycho-Oncology 2015;25(5):491–495. doi: 10.1002/pon.3945.

5. Wang YH, Li JQ, Shi JF, et al. Depression and anxiety in relation to cancer incidence and mortality: A systematic review and meta-analysis of cohort studies. Mol Psychiatry. 2020;25(7):1487–1499.

6. McFarland DC, Doherty M, Atkinson TM, et. al. Cancer-related inflammation and depressive symptoms: Systematic review and meta-analysis. Cancer. 2022; 128(13):2504–2519.

7. National Comprehensive Cancer Network. NCCN Clinical Practice Guideline Distress Management, version 1. 2025.

8. Vita G, Compri B, Matcham F, Barbui C, Ostuzzi G. Antidepressants for the treatment of depression in people with cancer. Cochrane Database Syst Rev. 2023;3(3):CD011006.

9. Andersen BL, Lacchetti C, Ashing K, et al. Management of anxiety and depression in adult survivors of cancer: ASCO guideline update. J Clin Oncol. 2023;41(18):3426–3453.

10. Grassi L, Caruso R, Riba MB, et. Al. ESMO Guidelines Committee. Anxiety and depression in adult cancer patients: ESMO Clinical Practice Guideline. ESMO Open. 2023;8(2):101155.

11. Chayadi E, Baes N, Kiropoulos L. The effects of mindfulness-based interventions on symptoms of depression, anxiety, and cancer-related fatigue in oncology patients: A systematic review and meta-analysis. PLoS One. 2022;17(7):e0269519.

12. Qin M, Chen B, Sun S, Liu X. Effect of mobile phone app-based interventions on quality of life and psychological symptoms among adult cancer survivors: Systematic review and meta-analysis of randomized controlled trials. J Med Internet Res. 2022;24(12): e39799.

13. Caruso R, Nanni M, Riba MB, Sabato S, Grassi L. Depressive spectrum disorders in cancer: Diagnostic issues and intervention. A critical review. Curr Psychiatry Rep. 2017;19(6):33.

14. Wakefield CE, Butow PN, Aaronson NA, et al. Patient-reported depression measures in cancer: A meta-review. Lancet Psychiatry. 2015;2(7):635–647.

15. Beck AT, Steer RA, Brown GK. Manual for the Beck Depression Inventory - Fast Screen for Medical Patients. Psychological Corporation, 2000.

16. Dils AT, O'Keefe K, Dakka N, Azar M, Chen M, Zhang A. The efficacy of cognitive behavioral therapy for mental health and quality of life among individuals diagnosed with cancer: A systematic review and meta-analysis. Cancer Med. 2024;13(16):e70063.

17. Uphoff E, Pires M, Barbui C, et.al. Behavioural activation therapy for depression in adults with non-communicable diseases. Cochrane Database Syst Rev. 2020;8(8):CD013461.

18. Hart SL, Hoyt MA, Diefenbach M, et al. Meta-analysis of efficacy of interventions for elevated depressive symptoms in adults diagnosed with cancer. J Natl Cancer Inst. 2012;104(13):990–1004.

19. Andrew BN, Guan NC, Jaafar NRN. The use of methylphenidate for physical and psychological symptoms in cancer patients: A review. Curr Drug Targets. 2018;19(8):877–887.

20. Dean RL, Hurducas C, Hawton K, et al. Ketamine and other glutamate receptor modulators for depression in adults with unipolar major depressive disorder. Cochrane Database Syst Rev. 2021;9(9):CD011612.

21. Schipper S, Nigam K, Schmid Y, et.al. Psychedelic-assisted therapy for treating anxiety, depression, and existential distress in people with life-threatening diseases. Cochrane Database Syst Rev. 2024;9(9):CD015383.

22. Carlson LE, Ismaila N, Addington EL, et.al. Integrative oncology care of symptoms of anxiety and depression in adults with cancer: Society for Integrative Oncology: ASCO guideline. J Clin Oncol. 2023;41(28):4562–4591.

23. Li M, Kennedy EB, Byrne N, et al. Systematic review and meta-analysis of collaborative care interventions for depression in patients with cancer. Psycho-Oncology. 2017;26(5):573–587.

Further Reading and Resources

Watson M, Kissane D, eds. *Management of Clinical Depression and Anxiety*. Oxford University Press; 2017.

An IPOS-supported set of guidelines for the management of anxiety and depression in cancer care.

Watson M, Kissane D, eds. *Handbook of Psychotherapy in Cancer Care*. Oxford University Press, 2nd ed.; 2026.

Comprehensive outline of the models of psychotherapy delivered in cancer care.

Chapter 5

Cancer Treatment-Related Cognitive Change

Joanne Fardell, Mu-Hsing Ho, Tim Ahles, and Janette Vardy

Learning Objectives

After reading this chapter, the clinician will be able to:

1. Understand the prevalence, risk, and presentation of cognitive difficulties among survivors of cancers diagnosed with non–central nervous system cancer who are older than 18 years.
2. Gain insight into how to identify cognitive difficulties among cancer survivors.
3. Know what evidence-based interventions are currently recommended for cancer survivors experiencing cognitive difficulties.

Background Evidence

This chapter focuses on cancer-related cognitive changes and symptoms in adults diagnosed with a non–central nervous system cancer and who are older than 18 years. Studies show that memory, processing speed, attention, and executive function (in particular aspects of attentional control such as shifting, updating, and/or working memory) are the cognitive domains most affected by chemotherapy.[1,2] For most people, the cognitive impairment is subtle, and they may still score within the normal range on neuropsychological tests. However, even subtle changes can be problematic, especially for those still working and those with a lifestyle with high cognitive demands.[3]

The cognitive sequelae of adults diagnosed with central nervous system (CNS) tumors are well described. This population experiences significant risk of profound cognitive impairment, personality change, mood disturbance, and physical limitations because of their brain tumor and its treatment. Survivors of brain cancer require multifaceted and multidisciplinary support and rehabilitation across many domains of functioning, and, as such, their specific needs will not be covered in this chapter.

Symptoms of cancer-related cognitive changes can occur in up to 80% of adults undergoing chemotherapy, with around 50% experiencing persistent cognitive symptoms due to their cancer and/or cancer treatment.[1,4,5]

Cognitive symptoms are consistently associated with fatigue, anxiety, depression, and poorer quality of life. However, these symptoms are only weakly associated with performance on formal neuropsychological testing. Neuropsychological assessment indicates that 30–45% of survivors of adult cancers have cognitive impairment months to years after receiving chemotherapy with curative intent, but the rates vary considerably based on the treatment, time since chemotherapy, and the definition of cognitive impairment used.[1] One study found cognitive difficulties persisting 20 years after chemotherapy.

Studies consistently show that up to 30% of individuals who never received chemotherapy or had not yet undergone surgery or systemic therapy may score lower than expected on neuropsychological testing.[1] The decline in cognitive function before treatment suggests tumor-derived factors may play a role in influencing cognition and behavior.[1] The exact cause of cognitive difficulties is not fully understood, with conflicting study results, but it is likely multifactorial.[6,7] These factors may include direct toxicity that affects the blood–brain barrier, complex interactions between inflammatory cytokines, genetic polymorphisms (e.g., apolipoprotein E [APOE] and catechol-o-methyltransferase [COMT], and brain-derived neurotrophic factor [BDNF]), DNA and mitochondrial damage, and psychosocial components (stress, anxiety, depression).[7]

Risk factors are not clearly defined but include chemotherapy, older age at the time of chemotherapy, and a lack of cognitive reserve.[8]

Neuroimaging studies have demonstrated that people who have undergone chemotherapy experience accelerated brain aging; a reduction in gray matter volume, particularly in frontal regions; and a decrease in white matter integrity. Functional magnetic resonance imaging (fMRI) has revealed hypoactivation in certain brain regions when performing some memory tasks compared to non-chemotherapy survivors and non-cancer controls.[1,9] Some studies have also found increased activity in other brain regions in chemotherapy-treated survivors compared to those who did not receive chemotherapy, with no difference in task performance, suggesting a compensatory mechanism to engage additional brain areas to maintain performance. Though there are other contributing factors, this may partially explain the lack of association between self-reported cognitive symptoms and cognitive impairment observed on neuropsychological assessment: survivors may be aware of working harder but use compensatory mechanisms to arrive at the correct answer (see Costa and Fardell [2019] for a discussion paper on why self-reported cognitive difficulties are poorly correlated with standardized neuropsychological assessments).[10]

A limitation worth acknowledging is that most of the research on the cognitive impacts of cancer and cancer treatment has been in women with breast cancer,[9,11] but studies have confirmed similar findings in men and in other solid and hematological tumor types. Endocrine therapies, particularly tamoxifen, immunotherapy, and targeted therapies, have also been shown to cause cognitive difficulties but are less well-researched.[1]

Presenting Problems

Key Symptoms and Signs

People typically describe problems with their memory, poor concentration, and difficulty multitasking. They often have trouble with word finding. These symptoms usually peak during chemotherapy and improve over time, but often do not fully resolve. Some people notice these issues when they return to work and realize they cannot function as well as before. For example, people may find themselves falling behind at work, unable to keep on top of tasks that they could previously manage, fail to complete tasks, and/or find themselves easily distracted and not completing a task before starting a new one. Tasks may take longer to complete and feel harder to do so. Many who self-report cognitive symptoms also experience fatigue, symptoms of anxiety and depression, distress, sleep disruption,[12] and a lower quality of life, so it is important to assess and treat these as needed.

Case Study 1

A 42-year-old premenopausal woman was diagnosed with early-stage breast cancer. Following a wide local excision and sentinel node biopsy, she underwent adjuvant chemotherapy with Adriamycin and cyclophosphamide (AC) followed by paclitaxel. She then received breast radiotherapy and started taking tamoxifen.

She provided a detailed account of experiencing worsening cognitive symptoms around the third cycle of chemotherapy. She specifically mentioned difficulty with word finding, forming sentences, and experiencing memory issues such as forgetting what she had read or done, misplacing objects, and struggling with multitasking. She was highly educated and held a demanding, high-level job, and she noted that several aspects of her work had become challenging. She expressed feeling anxious about these changes and a loss of confidence in her abilities.

She had discontinued tamoxifen about 6 months previously, initially temporarily when travelling, and noticed an improvement in her cognitive symptoms. She sought assistance due to concerns about maintaining her job.

Management

A neuropsychological assessment was suggested to determine if there was any objective cognitive impairment and, if so, which cognitive domains were most affected. While there are no good comparisons between different aromatase inhibitors, switching to exemestane was recommended because there is increasing evidence that tamoxifen has more cognitive side effects than exemestane, and she was now postmenopausal. Information and compensatory strategies were provided from a trusted website (see Resources below). Engaging in other activities like puzzles, learning a new activity (e.g., musical instrument, dancing, language), and exercise were encouraged. An online brain training program, previously trialed,[13] was suggested for 20 minutes three times a week. Although she did not have overt symptoms of depression, clinical psychology follow-up was recommended to help with adjustment to life after cancer.

Diagnosis and Assessment

The mismatch between cognitive symptoms self-reported on patient reported outcome measures (PROMs) and cognitive performance on standardized neuropsychological assessment, along with the co-occurrence of other symptoms that are known to impact cognitive function, can make diagnosis challenging (see below for a discussion of differential diagnosis considerations). Assessing for cognitive symptoms and their impact should ideally take the following step-wise approach:

- First, assess symptoms by asking directly about them (Box 5.1) or by using validated cognitive symptom PROMs (see Box 5.2).
- Second, where self-reported cognitive symptoms are frequent, severe, and impact functioning (e.g., ability to fulfil family and occupational roles or ability to study are impacted), and/or cognitive symptoms are associated with psychological distress, assessment for cognitive abilities and impairments using a neuropsychological assessment may be considered (see Box 5.3)

Cognitive screening tests, which involve brief assessment of cognitive skills and abilities, such as the Mini-Mental State Examination and Montreal Cognitive Assessment (MoCA) are designed to screen for dementia and are not suitable for identifying cancer-related cognitive impairment.[14] It is recommended to refer patients showing signs of cognitive impairment to a neuropsychologist for formal neuropsychological testing. The Fast Cognitive Evaluation (FaCE) has been developed recently as a screening tool for detecting cognitive impairment in cancer patients,[15] although further research is required.

Key Point

Assessing for cognitive symptoms using self-report is an important first step in assessment.

Box 5.1 Assessing Cognitive Symptoms through Self-Report

The following questions have been recommended by the National Comprehensive Cancer Network Guidelines on Survivorship (Version 2.2024) to help clarify the nature and impact of cognitive symptoms people with a history of cancer may experience:

- Do you have difficulty paying attention? Multitasking?
- Do you frequently leave tasks incomplete?
- Do you have difficulty finding words?
- Do you have difficulty remembering things?
- Do you need to use more prompts like notes or reminders than you used to?
- Does it take you longer to think through problems; does your thinking seem slower?
- Do you notice an impact on functional performance? Job performance?

Box 5.2 Patient-Reported Outcome Measures (PROMs)

These are surveys or questionnaires that measure outcomes that matter most to patients. These validated tools can be used to

- Assess the severity, frequency, and functional impacts of cognitive symptoms from the perspective of the patient,
- Provide important contextual information and information about the burden of cognitive symptoms from the perspective of the person with a history of cancer,
- Facilitate clinical discussions,
- Identify potential clinically meaningful and significant cognitive symptoms (based on published cutoff scores), and
- Inform development of cognitive strategies and intervention suggestions.

PROMs that have been developed and/or validated in oncology populations[16] include

- The Patient-Reported Outcomes Measurement Information System (PROMIS) Cognitive Function
- Functional Assessment of Cancer Therapy – Cognitive Function (FACT-Cog)
  Other PROMs that may be useful include
- Everyday Memory Questionnaire
- Patient's Assessment of Own Functioning Inventory (PAOFI)[16]

- However, it is important to note that self-report of symptoms is not a proxy for measurement of cognitive function due to the poor correlation between self-report of cognitive symptoms and cognitive function as measured by neuropsychological assessment.
- Selecting the appropriate PROMs to use should involve careful consideration of the availability of the normative sample used to generate the cutoff when interpreting individual PROM scores. Ideally the population used to generate the clinical cutoff score should match the age, sex, and diagnosis of the survivor completing the PROM.

🔍 Key Point

For psychologists assessing cognitive function it is important to establish the goals of undertaking a neuropsychological assessment, given the time and cost involved.

For example,

- establish an understanding of cognitive function and capacity after cancer treatment;
- identify strategies, recommendations, or interventions to remediate cognitive symptoms;
- support return to study or work; and
- establish new career goals in line with abilities and priorities after cancer.

Box 5.3 Neuropsychological Assessment

Neuropsychological assessment can only be conducted by a suitably qualified psychologist or neuropsychologist and involves

1. Conducting a thorough clinical interview and history and
2. Assessment of cognitive performance on standardized testing designed to specifically assess cognitive skills and abilities using both pencil-and-paper and computerized tests.

Duration of assessment can vary, sometimes taking up to several hours.

Considerations for the clinical interview and history-taking in the context of cancer survivorship include:

- Establishing the time course of cognitive symptoms, when they first occurred relative to cancer diagnosis and treatment, and any pre-cancer cognitive symptoms.
- Identification of any potential confounding and/or contributing factors (see "Investigations for Key Differential Diagnosis" section), especially fatigue and sleep and mood disturbances.

Considerations for cognitive assessment in the context of cancer survivorship include:

- In general, neuropsychological practice favors a flexible assessment—tests are chosen according to the patient's history and the referral question. But, in some instances, a battery approach (where the same tests are administered to every patient) is favored. At present, the tests that are most sensitive to impairment among people living with and beyond cancer is yet to be established clinically or empirically.
- Clinicians are encouraged to prioritize the assessment of domains previously shown to be impaired (i.e., memory, processing speed, attention/working memory, and executive function).
- Clinicians should consider an individual's specific needs and concerns, suitability of tests, availability of appropriate age and sex norms, and any needed cultural or language adaptations/requirements when selecting neuropsychological tests.
- The following battery of tests has been suggested by the International Cognition and Cancer Taskforce (ICCTF)[11] in an attempt to harmonize data collected through research studies:
  - Hopkins Verbal Learning Test-Revised (HVLT-R)
  - Trail Making Test (TMT)
  - Controlled Oral Word Association (COWA) of the Multilingual Aphasia Examination

Investigations for Key Differential Diagnoses

Key Differentials

- Resolution of symptoms including sleep disturbance, mental health concerns, fatigue, and pain prior to comprehensive neuropsychological assessment is ideal. These commonly occurring late effects after cancer are known contributors to reductions in cognitive function in the general population and can impact cognitive function in cancer populations.[1,3] Assessment shortly after chemotherapy treatment completion is not recommended due to the high prevalence of confounding symptoms, especially fatigue.[3]

- Consideration of specific treatment-related impacts such as changes to endocrine function subsequent to cancer treatment (e.g., diabetes, treatment-induced menopause, hypo- or hyperthyroidism), potential cardiotoxicity, neurotoxicity, and immune effector cell-associated neurotoxicity syndrome (ICANS) in the instance of targeted therapies, is warranted since these conditions can affect cognitive function.

- Evaluation of late toxicities of cancer treatments is particularly important when evaluating older, long-term survivors because studies have suggested that cognitive function is mediated by the accumulation of comorbidities and psychosocial and functional problems in older breast cancer survivors.[17]

- Differential diagnosis in older survivors of cancer (>75 years of age) should consider the potential for developing dementia versus cognitive difficulties as a result of cancer and/or its treatment.

- Potential contributing factors to cognitive function, including past medical history (e.g., past diagnosis of development or cognitive concerns, attention-deficit/hyperactivity disorder (ADHD), past head injuries, or serious illness and hospitalization), education history (e.g., level of academic achievement), and family history (e.g., diagnosis of dementia, psychological or psychiatric diagnoses), should be assessed (see Case Study 2).

- Lifestyle factors that confer cognitive risk in the general population, such as smoking, alcohol and drug intake, level of physical activity, diet, and level of social support and participation, should also be considered.

Case Study 2

A 74-year-old man with a history of prostate adenocarcinoma diagnosed 3 years earlier was referred by his oncologist for neuropsychological testing in the context of a 2-year history of reported cognitive changes. Reported cognitive changes included word-finding difficulties and trouble focusing, as well as symptoms of depression and fatigue since undergoing treatments including chemotherapy, radiation therapy, and androgen deprivation therapy. After consulting his oncologist, he discontinued leuprolide approximately 6 months ago. Since then, he reported significant improvement in depression and fatigue, facilitating a return to regular exercise and swimming, as well as "mental clearing." Word-finding difficulties and some memory difficulty persisted, and he needed "some help with business affairs." No changes in sensorimotor function, appetite, or sleep were observed. He wakes up three or four times a night to catheterize. He lives alone and reports full functional independence. He spends his time socializing, exercising regularly, and shopping.

Additional history includes hepatitis C, aneurysm, DVT, hypercholesterolemia, hyperlipidemia, coronary bypass surgery, stent placement (×3), appendectomy, bowel obstruction with lysis of adhesions, and cystoscopy and transurethral resection of bladder tumor. He reported remote history of concussion, without loss of consciousness, sustained playing football as a child. Long-standing depression, anxiety, and "emotional disturbance" as a child was reported, and he has continued to see a psychiatrist on and off since late adolescence.

At the time of the neuropsychological assessment, prescribed medications included bupropion, alfuzosin, tadalafil, pitavastatin, lisinopril, vitamin D, and montelukast.

Some early academic difficulty due to emotional disturbance and attention deficit disorder were reported. He went on to achieve an MA and PhD in finance and has worked in finance, real estate, and banking in various capacities in his career. He is widowed, lives alone, and has one son. He ceased working following diagnosis of his prostate cancer.

Management

With this history and presenting complaint as a context, a comprehensive neuropsychological evaluation was conducted that included standard measures of attention and working memory, processing speed, language, visuospatial ability, executive function, and learning and memory. Self-reported anxiety and depression were also assessed.

Premorbid cognitive abilities were estimated to be in the high average range, given educational and vocational attainment and performance on the evaluation that is indicative of lifetime cognitive abilities. Results suggested vulnerabilities in language and semantic fluency and select aspects of visual learning and memory in an otherwise normal profile. This pattern of results, including semantic fluency and word-finding difficulties, together with mild impairment in visual learning and recall, may suggest cognitive effects of treatment although it is noted that leuprolide has been discontinued for the past 6 months. At the same time, treatment history confers greater risk of cognitive difficulties, particularly given age at treatment and the duration of multiple treatments since diagnosis, along with several comorbidities that may independently increase risk of cognitive difficulties. Considered in the context of reported cognitive changes, his neurocognitive status warrants monitoring over time to track any prospective changes in ability, progression of difficulty, or decline in his ability to live and/or function independently.

Essential Tests and Further Assessment

Neuropsychological assessment (see Box 5.3) by a suitably qualified clinician is required to describe a survivor's cognitive profile of strengths, weaknesses, and any cognitive impairment. If available, review of magnetic resonance brain imaging (MRI) to identify other contributing factors such as infarcts or small-vessel disease can aid in interpreting the comprehensive neuropsychological assessment but is not required and is often not available to survivors (who have no evidence of CNS-disease) without incurring extensive out-of-pocket costs.

Clinical Management

Cognitive difficulties and symptoms present a significant challenge for people living with and beyond cancer, impacting their activities of daily living and quality of life. Table 5.1 provides an outline for recommended steps for survivorship care, highlighting areas for tailoring plans to the individual survivor's particular needs and circumstances.

Table 5.1 Recommendations for management of cognitive changes after cancer	
1.	*Assessment:*
	Regularly assess and detect cognitive function changes using validated tools for subjective (self-reported) cognitive complaints and objective cognitive performance. Consider and assess for the presence of other contributing factors and symptoms as a result of cancer treatment.
2.	*Provide support:*
	Normalize concerns about cognitive function and validate the impact cognitive symptoms have on day-to-day function. Provide information on relevant strategies for managing cognitive symptoms in the context of living with and after cancer (see "Further Resources"). For example, in the instance of memory difficulties, provide coaching and instruction on how to use phone reminders and calendars; or, where task tracking and attention difficulties are present, how to create task lists and monitor progress.
3.	*Individualized intervention plans:*
	Develop tailor-made plans that incorporate strategies/interventions based on specific cognitive challenges and individual preferences. Neuropsychological assessment can identify specific areas of cognitive weakness or difficulty and tailor strategies accordingly. Management plans and offered interventions should be considered in the context of the individual's current life circumstances and goals for assessment. For example, does the individual have the means and necessary support (financial, social) to act on the provided recommendations or suggested interventions?
4.	*Multidisciplinary approach:*
	Collaborate with specialists in psychology, rehabilitation, nutrition, nursing, and physical therapy to provide comprehensive care tailored to the survivors needs, taking a "whole-person" quality of life approach to addressing cognitive impairment.
5.	*Education:*
	Provide information to survivors about the potential benefits of treatments and the multifactorial nature of cognitive symptoms after cancer treatment. Encourage active participation in treatment decisions and consider changes or accommodations to current education or career goals consistent with the survivor's values and burden of cognitive symptoms.
6.	*Monitoring progress:*
	Continuously monitor survivor's cognitive function changes and quality of life through follow-up assessments to evaluate the effectiveness of interventions and make necessary adjustments.

Pharmacological Options

Pharmacological interventions for cognitive impairment have been explored along potential causal pathways.[18] Most research to date has focused on developing and testing, in rodent models, with cancer-related cognitive impairment, those antioxidants, antidepressants, and psychostimulants commonly used in the treatment of ADHD. However, current options remain limited. Evidence to date is often inconclusive, with few trials conducted with those living with and beyond cancer (see Rao et al. [2022] for a discussion of pharmacological interventions based on putative causal mechanisms[7]). There is insufficient evidence to recommend any pharmacological drug for use in non–CNS cancer-related cognitive change.

Nonpharmacological Interventions for Cancer-Related Cognitive Changes

Nonpharmacological interventions have emerged as important supportive strategies for managing cognitive difficulties. Recent network meta-analyses (NMAs) of randomized controlled trials evaluated the effectiveness of various aforementioned nonpharmacological interventions for cognitive difficulties among survivors of adult cancer without central nervous system involvement.[19,20] The results indicate that *cognitive training, rehabilitation, meditation/mindfulness-based interventions, and exercise* are among the most effective interventions for improving subjective cognitive function for people living with and beyond cancer. None of the studies reported significant adverse events associated with these interventions, suggesting they are safe options for managing cognitive changes after cancer. The findings from these NMAs highlight the importance of integrating nonpharmacological interventions into clinical practice for managing cognitive impacts experienced by people with a history of cancer.

Psychotherapeutic Approaches

- *Cognitive training*: Cognitive training involves structured exercises designed to enhance specific cognitive skills through practice. Typically employing computerized tasks, cognitive training focuses on retraining memory, attention, and executive functions. The tasks are tailored to increase in difficulty based on individual performance, allowing for personalized training.[20] Most cognitive training has targeted higher-order cognitive function. However, given increasing evidence that people with a history of cancer experience changes in early attentional control processes that support higher-order cognitive function (e.g., difficulty filtering irrelevant information and increased variability in attentional focus/mind wandering), several researchers have developed interventions designed to enhance "bottom-up" processes. Initial results are promising, particularly when combined with interventions designed to improve top-down cognitive processes.[21]

- *Cognitive rehabilitation*: Cognitive rehabilitation is a more comprehensive approach than cognitive training incorporating psychoeducation, skills training, and functional activity training. It aims to help individuals regain lost cognitive functions by applying learned strategies in everyday life. This intervention is particularly beneficial for those who have experienced significant cognitive decline due to cancer treatments.[19] Qualified psychologists and neuropsychologists are able to deliver cognitive rehabilitation, with offerings in both individual and group format.

- *Meditation/mindfulness-based interventions*: These practices focus on enhancing mental well-being through relaxation and increased awareness of the present moment. Meditation techniques often involve breath regulation and thought control, while some mindfulness-based stress reduction interventions emphasize sustaining attention on current experiences and cultivating an attitude of curiosity and acceptance.[20]

- *Cognitive behavioral therapy (CBT)*: CBT focuses on modifying negative thoughts that can exacerbate cognitive difficulties and emotional distress. By addressing these issues, CBT improves overall cognitive function and emotional resilience.[22]

- *Supportive therapy*: Interventions provide emotional support through consultation and discussions with healthcare professionals regarding health-related concerns and coping strategies. It encourages survivors to share their experiences and feelings in a safe environment. [20]

Lifestyle and Behavioral Approaches

- *Physical activity and exercise*: Regular physical activity is crucial for maintaining overall health and has been shown to improve cognitive function among people living with and beyond cancer. Interventions may include light movement, aerobic exercise, or moderate to vigorous exercise, all of which promote physical activity levels. Studies have consistently shown that aerobic exercise enhances blood flow to the brain while promoting neurogenesis, the formation of new neurons, which is essential for maintaining cognitive health post-cancer treatment. Current National Comprehensive Cancer Network (NCCN) physical activity guidelines recommend that survivors aim to engage in at least 150 minutes of weekly activity with an ultimate goal of 300 minutes or more of moderate-intensity activity or 75 minutes of vigorous-intensity activity or equivalent combination spread out over the course of the week (see "Further Reading and Resources").

- *Traditional Chinese medicine-based interventions*:
  - *Acupuncture/acupoint stimulation*: A technique that balances yin/yang and qi/blood by stimulating specific locations (acupoints) along the body's meridians with various stimulation methods such as needling (acupuncture) and pressure (acupressure).
  - *Tai chi and Qigong*: These mind–body practices originating in China are studied for their effectiveness in stress reduction and symptom management through meditative movements.[20]

- *New and emerging therapeutic interventions*:
  - *Transcranial direct current stimulation (tDCS)*: tDCS is a noninvasive technique that modulates neural activity in the brain by delivering low-amplitude stimulation through the scalp. Proposed mechanisms of

action include modulation of neurotransmitter activity and increase in neuroplasticity and connectivity. Two small studies suggest that tDCS applied to frontal regions improves executive function and attention.[23] Combining cognitive training with tDCS is a promising area for future study.

Professional Issues and Service Implementation

Recording and Communicating

Local and national professional accreditation and practice standards should be followed with regard to documenting the occurrence of cognitive symptoms. At a minimum, when survivors report cognitive symptoms during a clinical encounter, these should be recorded in relevant electronic medical records, with an action plan and follow-up plan noted. Given the potential for distress in any clinical encounter, survivors should be offered a written summary of the issues discussed and suggested management plan, including self-management cognitive strategies. Widespread implementation of patient portals within electronic medical records will ultimately support communicating back results and suggested cognitive strategies and management plans with survivors.

Common Ethical Dilemmas

Access to comprehensive neuropsychological assessment and cognitive rehabilitation services may be challenging for some survivors due to local resourcing, their care delivery setting (e.g., private and public health services), and their level of insurance coverage. Additionally, comprehensive neuropsychological assessment may not be warranted in all cases. Given the burden of such assessments (practically, financially, and time required), careful consideration should be given to referral to neuropsychology. A thorough clinical interview conducted by a suitably qualified clinician (psychologist) may provide sufficient information to generate supportive strategies for people living with cognitive symptoms in the first instance.

Cognitive symptoms can have a significant impact on day-to-day functioning, especially in the context of returning to study or work. As such, when survivors report cognitive difficulties that are impacting quality of life and ability to fulfil roles, supportive interventions (especially those with reasonable evidence reviewed above, such as cognitive training, rehabilitation, meditation/mindfulness-based interventions, and exercise) should be offered. Clinicians conducting assessments (whether using clinical interviews, PROMs, or neuropsychological tests) should carefully consider likely pre-cancer cognitive function to determine specific cognitive challenges a survivor may be experiencing to support the development of tailored cognitive strategies and interventions.

Teams and Supervision

Given that the cause of cognitive symptoms after cancer can be multifactorial and the subsequent management of cognitive symptoms may be multidisciplinary, ensuring that teams responsible for survivorship care contain health professionals spanning medical, nursing, exercise physiology and psychology (including neuropsychology) will support delivery of best-practice care for survivors.

Ongoing supervision for psychologists and neuropsychologists is a requirement for accreditation/licensing in almost all countries and should be adhered to. However, given the rapid increase in the number of research studies investigating cancer-related cognitive changes and possible interventions, clinicians will benefit from continuing professional development activities that support engaging with this emerging research.

Acknowledgments

Joanna Fardell is a Maridulu Budyari Gumal (SPHERE) Cancer CAG Senior Research Fellow and is supported by a Cancer Institute NSW Research Capacity Building Grant (2021/CBG003)

Mu-Hsing Ho is supported by the Health and Medical Research Fund (HMRF), Research Fellowship Scheme (Project No. 08220207), Health Bureau, the government of the Hong Kong Special Administrative Region.

Tim Ahles is supported by grants from the National Cancer Institute (TA: R01 CA276265, R01 CA240417 U54 CA137788, P30 CA008748).

Janette Vardy is supported by a National Health Medical Research Council Investigator Grant [APP1176221]

References

1. Lange M, Joly F, Vardy J, et al. Cancer-related cognitive impairment: An update on state of the art, detection, and management strategies in cancer survivors. Ann Oncol. 2019;30:1925–1940.

2. Yao C, Bernstein LJ, Rich JB. Executive functioning impairment in women treated with chemotherapy for breast cancer: A systematic review. Breast Cancer Res Treatm. 2017;166:15–28.

3. Fardell JE, Tan SYC, Kerin-Ayres K, et al. Symptom clusters in survivorship and their impact on ability to work among cancer survivors. Cancers (Basel). 2023;15(21):5119.

4. Fleming B, Edison P, Kenny L. Cognitive impairment after cancer treatment: Mechanisms, clinical characterization, and management. BMJ. 2023;380:e071726.

5. Demos-Davies K, Lawrence J, Seelig D. Cancer related cognitive impairment: A downside of cancer treatment. Front Oncol. 2024;14:1387251.

6. Ahles TA, Root JC. Cognitive effects of cancer and cancer treatments. Annu Rev Clin Psychol. 2018;14:435–451.

7. Rao V, Bhushan R, Kumari P, Cheruku SP, Ravichandiran V, Kumar N. Chemobrain: A review on mechanistic insight, targets and treatments. Adv Cancer Res. 2022;155:29–76.

8. Mohamed M, Ahmed M, Williams ALM, et al. A scoping review evaluating physical and cognitive functional outcomes in cancer survivors treated with

chemotherapy: Charting progress since the 2018 NCI think tank on cancer and aging phenotypes. J Survivorship. 2024. https://doi.org/10.1007/s11 764-024-01589-0

9. de Ruiter MB, Deardorff RL, Blommaert J, et al. Brain gray matter reduction and premature brain aging after breast cancer chemotherapy: A longitudinal multicenter data pooling analysis. Brain Imaging Behav. 2023;17:507–518.

10. Costa DSJ, Fardell JE. Why are objective and perceived cognitive function weakly correlated in patients with cancer? J Clin Oncol. 2019;37(14):1154–1158. doi: 10.1200/JCO.18.02363. Epub 2019 Mar 28. PMID: 30920881.

11. Wefel JS, Vardy J, Ahles T, et al. International Cognition and Cancer Task Force recommendations to harmonise studies of cognitive function in patients with cancer. Lancet Oncol. 2011;12:703–708.

12. Drijver AJ, Oort Q, Otten R, et al. Is poor sleep quality associated with poor neurocognitive outcome in cancer survivors? A systematic review. J Cancer Surviv. 2024;18:207–222.

13. Von Ah D, Crouch A, Storey S. Acceptability of computerized cognitive training and global cognitive stimulating-based games delivered remotely: Results from a randomized controlled trial to address cancer and cancer-related cognitive impairment in breast cancer survivors. Cancer Med. 2023;12:12717–12727.

14. Arcuri GG, Palladini L, Dumas G, et al. Exploring the measurement properties of the Montreal Cognitive Assessment in a population of people with cancer. Support Care Cancer. 2015;23:2779–2787.

15. Baghdadli A, Arcuri GG, Green CG, et al. The Fast Cognitive Evaluation (FaCE): A screening tool to detect cognitive impairment in patients with cancer. BMC Cancer. 2023;23:35.

16. Fardell JE, Bray V, Bell ML, et al. Screening for cognitive symptoms among cancer patients during chemotherapy: Sensitivity and specificity of a single item self-report cognitive change score. Psychooncology. 2022;31:1294–1301.

17. Ahles TA, Schofield E, Li Y, et al. Cognitive function is mediated by deficit accumulation in older, long-term breast cancer survivors. J Cancer Surviv. 2024;18:1243–1251.

18. Fardell JE, Vardy J, Johnston IN, et al. Chemotherapy and cognitive impairment: treatment options. Clin Pharmacol Ther. 2011;90:366–376.

19. Cheng ASK, Wang X, Niu N, et al. Neuropsychological interventions for cancer-related cognitive impairment: A network meta-analysis of randomized controlled trials. Neuropsychol Rev. 2022;32:893–905.

20. Zeng Y, Dong J, Huang M, et al. Nonpharmacological interventions for cancer-related cognitive impairment in adult cancer patients: A network meta-analysis. Int J Nurs Stud. 2020;104:103514.

21. Maeir T, Makranz C, Peretz T, et al. Cognitive Retraining and Functional Treatment (CRAFT) for adults with cancer related cognitive impairment: A preliminary efficacy study. Support Care Cancer. 2023;31:152.

22. Oldacres L, Hegarty J, O'Regan P, et al. Interventions promoting cognitive function in patients experiencing cancer related cognitive impairment: A systematic review. Psychooncology. 2023;32:214–228.

23. Gaynor AM, Pergolizzi D, Alici Y, et al. Impact of transcranial direct current stimulation on sustained attention in breast cancer survivors: Evidence for feasibility, tolerability, and initial efficacy. Brain Stimul. 2020;13:1108–1116.

Further Reading and Resources

Australia

Cancer Council. Changes in thinking and memory – with fact sheet https://www.cancer.org.au/cancer-information/cancer-side-effects/changes-in-thinking-and-memory

Hong Kong

Cancer Fund – Cancer Educational Videos: Chemo Brain. https://www.cancer-fund.org/en/cancer-videos/

Hong Kong Anti-Cancer Society – Cancer Info. Cancer Booklet. https://www.hkacs.org.hk/en/medicalnews.php?id=115

United States

National Cancer Institute. Home page. https://www.cancer.gov/about-cancer/treatment/side-effects/memory/cognitive-impairment-hp-pdq

National Comprehensive Cancer Network (NCCN). See NCCN Clinical Practice Guidelines in Oncology (NCCN Guidelines®) Survivorship Version 2.2024 — December 9, 2024 NCCN.org NCCN Guidelines for Patients. www.nccn.org/patients

https://www.nccn.org/patients/guidelines/content/PDF/survivorship-crl-patient.pdf

Chapter 6

Caregiver, Partner, and Family-Centered Support

Youngmee Kim and Kelly R. Tan

Learning Objectives

After reading this chapter, the clinician will be able to

1. Identify potential unmet needs of family caregivers and be cognizant of the impact on their health and well-being.
2. Gain knowledge about how to assess the unmet needs of family caregivers and detect subsequent psychosocial problems.
3. Acquire knowledge of current evidence-based therapies and national and international standards of resources to mitigate these unmet needs and psychosocial problems.

Background Evidence

Individuals with cancer have reported unmet needs that are primarily related to managing psychological distress, obtaining relevant information for cancer care, accomplishing daily activities, and dealing with physical symptoms and side effects of cancer treatment.[1] Family members and close friends of individuals with cancer (i.e., cancer caregivers) have also reported similar kinds of unmet needs and downstream psychological health problems when providing care and managing their own concerns due to the impact of cancer on the family and themselves throughout survivorship and bereavement. Unmet needs can lead to downstream effects on psychological health including increased risk for anxiety, depression, and sleep disturbance. In a meta-analysis of 30 studies, the prevalence estimate of anxiety was 46.6% and depression was 42.3% among cancer caregivers.[2]

In a nationwide study in the United States, caregivers reported encountering the greatest unmet need in managing psychological distress stemming from the individual with cancer, other family members, and themselves (>55%). Unmet needs related to the management of psychological distress are then followed by unmet needs related to obtaining proper medical care and symptom management for the patients (about 45%) and dealing with the caregivers' own personal care and balancing the caregiver role with other social roles (about 40%). Approximately one-third of caregivers (28%)

reported their need to manage financial concerns not being met.[3] According to Need Fulfillment Theory,[4] an unmet need is determined by the discrepancy between the importance of the need and satisfaction with how the need has been fulfilled. Such theory-driven operationalization underscores the critical roles of recognizing family caregivers' unmet needs by themselves, their other family members, and healthcare professionals as well as providing equitable access to programs and services that help fulfill these unmet needs.[5,6]

Caregivers' unmet needs typically decrease as the time since the patient's diagnosis increases; however, the prevalence of endorsing each of the diverse types of unmet needs varies based on the care recipient's current situation in relation to their cancer trajectory (e.g., diagnosis, active treatment, survivorship, bereavement). For example, at the time of diagnosis and treatment initiation, helping the patient's emotional distress, getting information about the cancer the patient was diagnosed with, talking to the patient about their concerns, getting the best possible care for the patient, and dealing with lifestyle changes were the most frequently endorsed needs.[3] On the other hand, about 5 years into survivorship, dealing with the survivor's emotional distress, being satisfied with the caregiver's relationship with the survivor, understanding/navigating medical and/or insurance coverage, having enough insurance coverage for the survivor, and dealing with the caregiver's own emotional distress were the most frequently endorsed unmet needs.[3]

Family and Caregiving in the Context of Cancer

Family, close friends, and caregiving relationships vary greatly depending on family structures, cancer progression, and the overall health of the person with cancer. Several notable situations include when one individual provides care to one or more individuals with cancer; when an adolescent or young adult cares for their parent or grandparent with cancer; when an individual with cancer provides care to another family member with a disability or chronic illness or a young child; and when an individual is caring for their partner with cancer and their children. Each of these scenarios may lead to different unmet needs and experiences.

Cancer caregivers' experiences vary also depending on the patient's disease trajectory. Some caregivers may provide care for many continuous years in cases of metastatic disease or for long-term treatment side effects, whereas others intermittently disengage and re-engage in care with recurrences of cancer and others exit their caregiving role once the patient is in remission or no longer experiences any symptoms. Most caregivers cease their role within 5 years. During the period of cancer survivorship when the cancer is in remission, however, caregivers may continue to have psychological problems related to fear of cancer recurrence. Furthermore, about one-third are likely to re-engage in caregiving 5–10 years after the initial diagnosis due to disease progression or new cancer occurrence. Such changes in caregivers' status regarding the patients' survivorship have impacts on caregivers' unmet needs. For example, either prolonged caregiving or having a break from caregiving only to be followed by bereavement during long-term survivorship was related to various kinds of caregivers' unmet needs several years after the initial diagnosis of patients' cancer. Greater perceived caregiving stress during the earlier phase of survivorship also predicted all kinds of unmet needs several years later.[7] Those dealing with familial cancer may also have distinct unmet needs.

These findings emphasize the necessity of periodic assessment of caregiver status that may change throughout long-term survivorship. The findings also urge the provision of continuity of care into bereavement and the development of interventions and programs for cancer caregivers that are cognizant of patterns of caregiving passage and the distinct unmet needs of those caregivers. Such interventions and programs are likely to yield reduced unmet needs and improved quality of life of family caregivers.

Presenting Problems

These various unmet needs of caregivers substantially predicted caregivers' mental and physical health. For example, caregivers whose psychosocial needs were not being met reported poorer mental health, such as elevated anxiety, depression, and cognitive confusion, consistently and strongly across different survivorship phases. Additionally, other types of unmet needs associated with poorer mental health at different phases of survivorship included medical unmet needs at the early survivorship phase, daily activity unmet needs at the early and mid-term survivorship phases, and financial unmet needs at mid- and long-term survivorship phases.[3]

Regarding the physical health of the caregivers, financial unmet needs, such as the unmet needs for taking care of bills, having enough insurance coverage for the survivor, and paying for the survivor's medical expenses were related to poorer physical health such as daily functioning and sleep problems at the early and mid-term phases of the survivorship. These findings highlight the importance of assessing caregivers' unmet needs, access to care, and particularly the mental health and financial burden involved in cancer care. It is vital to assess how these issues affect family caregivers' quality of life beyond treatment phases, with special emphasis on preventing disease in family caregivers.[3]

Another point worth noting is that caregivers' unmet needs became weak predictors of their quality of life several years after the cancer diagnosis of a relative, whereas demographic characteristics remained as strong predictors. Specifically, older age, female gender, and less education and income were risk factors for caregivers' poorer mental and physical health. These findings suggest that attention should be given to identifying subgroups of caregivers who are more likely to have greater unmet needs and be vulnerable to compromised quality of life. Those subgroups should be the focus of patient- and caregiver-centered care policies and prioritized to receive evidence-based programs through which their unmet needs can be mitigated.[3,7]

Cumulative psychosocial issues associated with caregiving can lead to or exacerbate psychiatric diagnoses. The primary diagnoses of concern include adjustment disorders, generalized anxiety disorder, depressive disorders, post-traumatic stress disorder (PTSD), and insomnia disorder.

Case Study

Juliana, a 34-year-old marketing manager, became the primary caregiver for her partner, Casey, after she was diagnosed with stage III colon cancer. They have two children: a 10-year-old son and a 7-year-old daughter. Upon hearing Casey's diagnoses, Juliana was initially shocked and in disbelief because Casey had always been the active and healthy one. Juliana had no idea how she was going to manage without Casey.

Casey's treatment included having part of her colon surgically removed and a 6-month course of FOLFOX adjuvant chemotherapy. Casey's surgery was uncomplicated, but her pain was poorly controlled. Juliana took a few days off work for Casey's surgery to do her best to manage Casey's pain but often felt powerless. Seven weeks after the surgery, Casey started her chemotherapy treatments. Everything was new to the family: the children struggled to find a new normal without Casey being available to drive them to their activities. Juliana struggled to juggle her job, caring for her children, and managing Casey's care. Juliana's company was supportive at first, but, due to a few missed deadlines, Juliana received disciplinary action. Juliana described each day as exhausting, overwhelming, unpredictable; she endorsed having anxiety and trouble sleeping.

Halfway through Casey's treatment, Juliana received the first of many medical bills. She spent many late evenings trying to figure out how they would be able to afford Casey's treatment, their mortgage, and basic living expenses. Although Juliana was getting the hang of caregiving tasks, the physical, psychological, and financial demands of caregiving took a toll on her mental health. Juliana was experiencing less anxiety about Casey's cancer but more anxiety about the family's financial issues, feeling hopeless and sad.

Two years after completing treatment, as the family began rebuilding, Casey's cancer aggressively returned and metastasized. Juliana quickly resumed her caregiving role, but she felt angry and frustrated that the life she had imagined for herself was nothing like her actual life. Casey received additional but unsuccessful treatment. Juliana was full of guilt, knowing that Casey wanted to be fully resuscitated but could not see how she would survive. Casey died a few days later when her heart stopped. After Casey's death, Juliana grieved. She missed Casey but was also relieved that she was no longer in pain. She felt angry at Casey for dying so suddenly and felt overwhelmed by sadness when she thought about their children.

Investigations for Key Differential Diagnoses

Several tools are available to screen for risk or general caregiving-related distress (see Table 6.1). Risk assessments can help identify caregivers with the highest risk for future psychosocial problems, whereas a distress screening tool measures current psychosocial issues. These tools are not diagnostic but can guide decision-making around further connecting caregivers to additional resources or further diagnoses of psychiatric conditions. Distress screening can be conducted by nonlicensed as well as licensed personnel (e.g., nurses, certified medical assistants, social workers, physicians, and psychologists);

Table 6.1 Screening tools and guidelines for detecting caregivers psychosocial issues

Psychosocial issue/diagnosis	Screening tool/ diagnostic guideline	# of items	Cancer caregiving specific considerations
Risk for caregiving-related issues.	Risk assessment screening tool[10]	16	Screening tool used to identify caregivers at highest risk for future issues across five domains (caregiving intensity, physical setting, care recipient suffering, social support, and caregiver's health)
Caregiving distress	Distress Screening tool[11]	18	Screening tool used to identify problem areas across six domains (practical, social/family, spiritual, information and skills, emotional, physical) Not to be used as a diagnostic tool. Identified problems should be followed-up with specific screeners and diagnostic tools, and/or appropriate resources.
Financial toxicity	Modified Comprehensive Score for Financial Toxicity[12]	11	Assessment of impact of cost of cancer treatment and caregiving on financial toxicity.
Caregiving burden	Caregiver Reaction Assessment[13]	24	Assesses perceived burden across 5 domains (impact on schedule, impact on finances, lack of family support, impact on health and self-esteem.
Fear of cancer recurrence	Fear of Cancer Recurrence Inventory-Short Form Caregiver Version[14]	9	Assessment of fear, worry, or concern relating to the possibility that cancer will come back or progress.
Adjustment disorders	DSM-5-TR[8]	--	The stressor(s) may be related to caregiving responsibilities and/or cancer related experiences.
Anxiety symptoms	Hospital Anxiety Depression Scale-Anxiety[15]	7	Generalized symptoms of anxiety and fear. Scores greater than 11 indicate moderate to severe anxiety symptoms and may warrant additional diagnostic follow-up
Generalized anxiety disorder	DSM-5-TR[8]	--	Anxiety and worry that extends beyond normal worry related to cancer or caregiving responsibilities.

Table 6.1 Continued

Psychosocial issue/diagnosis	Screening tool/ diagnostic guideline	# of items	Cancer caregiving specific considerations
Depressed mood	Patient Health Questionnaire (PHQ-9)[16]	9	General symptoms of depressed mood. Scores greater than 10 indicate moderate to severe depressive symptoms and may warrant additional diagnostic follow-up.
Depressive disorder	DSM-5-TR[8]	--	Depressive symptoms should not be better accounted for by cancer related bereavement.
Sleep disturbance	Brief-Pittsburgh Sleep Quality Index[17]	6	General assessment of sleep quality in the past month. Scores greater than 5 indicate poor sleep quality.
Sleep disorders – insomnia disorder	DSM-5-TR[8]	--	Difficulty sleeping or staying asleep may be related to actual caregiving tasks or emotional effects of caregiving.
Complicated grief/ bereavement/ prolonged grief disorder	Texas revised Inventory of complicated grief[18]	13	Assessment of pathological grief symptoms (e.g., anger, disbelief, and hallucinations).
Post-traumatic stress disorder	DSM-5-TR[8]	--	Traumatic event can be related to witnessing actual or threatened death of the person with cancer or prolonged exposure to aftereffects of death.

See DSM-5-TR[8] and diagnostic checklist for each diagnosis for more information.

however, a plan for follow-up for high distress should be in place prior to initiating distress screening in the clinical setting. After initial distress screening, further specific screening for individual psychological symptoms (e.g., anxiety, depression, sleep disturbance) may be warranted. In cases of persistent or severe distress, psychological symptoms, or referral (e.g., self- or oncology clinician), subsequent psychiatric diagnosis may be warranted. See also the most recent edition of the *Diagnostic and Statistical Manual of Mental Disorders* for specific criteria for commonly diagnosed disorders (e.g., adjustment disorders and depressive disorders) among caregivers.[8]

In some cases, caregivers may develop a host of psychological symptoms (e.g., anxiety, pain, sleep disturbance, flashbacks) because of repeated exposure to patient-related events (e.g., watching a person with cancer have a prolonged dying process with uncontrolled pain), the experience of a single traumatic event (e.g., watching the person with cancer receive cardiopulmonary resuscitation), or because of their own pre-existing issues not directly pertaining to cancer. In combination, these symptoms can be referred to as *acute stress disorder* or *post-traumatic stress* symptoms. Post-traumatic stress and PTSD may develop during the bereavement period after the person with cancer has died and caregiving responsibilities have ended. When caregiving roles end or are paused due to disease remission, individuals who had caregiving responsibilities continue to have psychological impacts related to cancer survivorship. During bereavement, caregivers go through grief processing, which can be uncomplicated or complicated. Normal *uncomplicated grief* involves a mix of persistent negative emotions and positive feelings that progressively improve over time. *Complicated grief* is characterized by intense, prolonged grief that impairs work, health, and social functioning, does not resolve, and may involve prolonged feelings of anger, intense loss, insomnia, and hallucinations. During bereavement, the terms "complicated grief" and "post-traumatic stress" can be used synonymously. Bereavement-specific distress can be assessed along with more general distress measures.[8] When caregiving roles pause due to disease remission caregivers may experience fear related to cancer recurrence.[9] From a meta-analysis of 45 studies, the prevalence of caregivers experiencing clinically significant fear of cancer recurrence was 48%.[9]

Clinical Management

Psychological Therapies

Both psychosocial issues that do not meet clinical diagnostic criteria (psychological symptoms) and those meeting clinical diagnostic criteria for psychological disorders can be addressed using pharmacologic and nonpharmacologic interventions. Note that these guidelines are not limited to caregivers. In some cases, a combination of the two types may be appropriate. Pharmacologic interventions should follow best practices for each psychiatric disorder. However, some caregivers without a psychiatric diagnosis may benefit from pharmacologic intervention for elevated levels of depressive and/or anxiety symptoms. The most prescribed medications for adjustment disorders, anxiety disorders/symptoms, and depressive disorders/symptoms are selective serotonin reuptake inhibitors (SSRIs) or serotonin norepinephrine reuptake inhibitors (SNRIs).[19]

Nonpharmacologic interventions are recommended for low, moderate, and severe distress because of their efficacy in improving psychological symptoms (see Table 6.2). Common no-pharmacologic interventions are general psychosocial support, supportive care interventions, skills-based interventions, and individual psychotherapy. Caregivers can benefit from general psychosocial support from individuals who interact with them in the care setting (e.g., clinicians, nurses, staff, social workers) and the daily setting (e.g., family and friends). Caregivers may also benefit from peer support through caregiving support groups where they can share and learn from other caregivers. The evidence base for caregiver support groups is limited, and the content and context of these groups is also highly variable. General psychosocial support includes recognizing individuals as caregivers, acknowledging their role, and providing emotional support through active listening and empathy when interacting with them.

Table 6.2 Evidence-based psychosocial interventions for cancer caregivers

Type of psychosocial intervention	Examples	Most appropriate for caregiver distress level	Time in cancer trajectory
General psychosocial support	Compassionate communication Information giving (local and national resources)	Any level	Throughout
Protocolized resource referral and social support	CancerSupportSource-Caregiver Caregiver Advocacy, Research, and Education Center	Any level	Treatment phase
Support programs	Structured group psychotherapy Unstructured support group.	Low to moderate	Throughout
Skills-based	Coping Strategies Social support interventions Positive Psychology Activities Mindfulness or Meditation Communication skills Problem-solving	Low to moderate	Treatment phase
Individual psychotherapy	Cognitive behavioral therapy Acceptance and Commitment Therapy Emotion Regulation Therapy for Caregivers Meaning Centered Psychotherapy for Caregivers Eye movement Desensitization and Reprocessing	Moderate to high	Treatment Phase, Post-treatment Phase

General Supportive Care Interventions

General supportive care interventions focus on systematically identifying distressed caregivers, providing support, and increasing access to existing resources and social networks. We highlight two protocolized supportive care interventions that can be broadly implemented because each intervention has demonstrated its efficacy: CancerSupportSource-Caregiver (CSS-C)[11] and Caregiver Advocacy, Research, and Education (CARE) Center.[10]

CSS-C is a distress screening, referral, and support program. CSS-C involves administering a 33-item electronic distress screener to caregivers that is then scored as overall distress and depression risk.[11] Caregivers are then automatically sent a report and access to educational materials. Caregivers who screen positive for distress or depression risk are followed-up by a licensed clinical psychologist. CSS-C has demonstrated moderate efficacy in improving emotional well-being.[11]

The CARE Center protocol also involves identification of caregivers, assessment of distress and unmet needs, and follow-up of distressed caregivers (those scoring >7 on the distress screener) by center staff who provide evidence-based self-management guides, self-management support, and referral to specialty services.[10] Both interventions address unmet needs, increase delivery of tailored support, and increase access to follow-up care for psychosocial issues.

Psycho-Educational and Skills-Based Interventions

Caregivers experiencing low to moderate distress mainly due to their recently acquired new role may also benefit from skills-based interventions that improve specific symptom management skills, stress management skills, and coping behavior skills. Skills-based interventions focus on providing psychoeducation and structured practice for specific coping behavior skills, communication skills, and/or problem-solving skills to reduce or manage caregiving-related stress. These interventions are typically delivered by a trained interventionist or clinician. Several recent meta-analyses concluded that skills-based interventions, specifically psychoeducational and problem-solving interventions, had moderate efficacy in improving anxiety and depression.[20] Increasingly, these interventions have been transitioned to web- or application-based delivery mode, and these modes are actively being studied.[21] Although these modes may address challenges in timing and access to interventions for caregivers, internet access and digital literacy should be taken into consideration.[21]

Skills-based interventions comprise a wide array of interventions including but not limited to social support interventions, coping behavior skills, and problem-solving interventions.[22] Social support interventions assist caregivers in identifying and accessing their own existing social support resources (e.g., family and friends who can help with caregiving tasks or other life responsibilities).[23] A key limitation of social support interventions is that caregivers with the highest distress may have limited access to social resources due to their life situation (e.g., family conflict, distance from other families).

Coping behavior skills interventions include positive psychology-based skills that focus on increasing caregivers' experiences of positive emotions in day-to-day life and stress reduction and management skills. Examples of positive psychology-based skills include gratitude journaling, finding moments of positivity, and loving kindness meditation.[24] Positive psychology-based interventions should be carefully delivered, recognizing that experienced negative emotions should not be minimized with simplistic optimism. Instead, positive psychology interventions provide an additional tool to cope with caregiving-related stress. Other coping behavior skills that can be improved include mindfulness, yoga, relaxation, and taking time for oneself.

Problem-solving skills can also be taught and involve instructing caregivers in how to identify and define problems, brainstorm potential solutions, make decisions and plans, and implement and evaluate solutions to caregiving-related problems.

Individual Psychotherapy

Caregivers experiencing moderate to high distress and caregivers with a psychiatric diagnosis likely benefit most from individualized support including one-on-one psychotherapy and more frequent follow-up. Individual in-person or telehealth psychotherapy can include therapies typically used for each psychiatric diagnosis; however, we focus here on four types of psychotherapy that have been tested in caregivers: (1) acceptance and commitment therapy (ACT),[25-27] (2) emotion regulation therapy (ERT-C),[28] (3) meaning-centered psychotherapy (MCP-C),[29] and (4) eye movement desensitization and reprocessing (EMDR).[30] All four types of psychotherapy are manualized, time-limited, and require additional training for their delivery.

- *ACT* is a type of cognitive behavioral therapy that focuses on caregivers learning to accept that feelings are appropriate responses to caregiving-related situations, undertake values-based behavior change, and develop psychological flexibility. ACT was found to have moderate effectiveness in reducing depressive symptoms and stress, improve quality of life, and exhibit small effects on anxiety in caregivers.[25,26] ACT may be better suited to address adjustment disorder, depressive disorders, and some anxiety disorders.

- *ERT-C* combines components of acceptance, mindfulness-based, emotion-focused, and cognitive behavioral treatments. ERT-C aims for caregivers to be able to differentiate their emotions, reduce perseverative negative thinking (e.g., worry, self-criticism), and increase acceptance of emotional experiences through skills training. ERT-C consists of eight weekly sessions with corresponding take-home exercises. Sessions cover specific emotion regulation skills such as self-monitoring, distancing, and courageous/compassionate reframing. ERT-C showed moderate to large effects in reducing psychological distress, burden, and depression and anxiety symptoms among cancer caregivers.[28]

- *MCP-C* focuses on helping caregivers find meaning and purpose despite experiencing caregiving challenges.[29] MCP-C may be particularly helpful for caregivers experiencing existential distress (e.g., feelings of regret, loss of personal meaning, and hopelessness). Caregivers receiving MCP-C are guided to reconnect with four sources of meaning in caregiving, including historical, attitudinal, creative, and experiential. Historical sources of meaning refer to past positive experiences of caregiving, achievements in the current caregiving role, and setting an example for future generations. MCP-C has shown preliminary efficacy in improving personal meaning and reducing depression symptoms.[29]

- *EMDR* focuses on changing the emotions, thoughts, or behaviors that result from a traumatic event or situation; in this case, caregiving-related trauma or complicated grief. EMDR works by helping caregivers form new associations with traumatic memories through desensitization and reprocessing of traumatic memories. EMDR typically is administered to the caregiver in six to eight sessions. EMDR has been shown to be effective in treating complicated grief and PTSD in caregivers.[30]

Professional Issues and Service Implementation

Recording and Communicating

Researchers and clinicians should assess the extent to which caregivers' needs are not being met using standardized assessment tools.[3] Furthermore, researchers and clinicians should also be cognizant that less-educated and ethnic/sexual minority caregivers as well as those whose cancer patients have more fatal types of initial diagnosis are often reluctant to vocalize their unmet needs. They are also less likely to participate in research studies involved in the assessment of unmet needs, which negatively affects the development and implementation of effective services that are critical to resolve these caregivers' needs. Special efforts to be inclusive to these underserved populations in research and clinical practice are important for providing equitable healthcare in which all family cancer caregivers' unmet needs are mitigated and their long-term quality of life is assured.

Clarify Referrals

Researchers and clinicians should refer to the list of screening tools and guidelines presented in Table 6.1 when making referrals for caregivers with psychosocial issues.

Legal Responsibilities

Reimbursement for services provided is evolving, but most commonly relies on consultation codes used for individual psychotherapy. These codes can only be used by licensed mental health professionals; however, provision of support to caregivers is also given by nonlicensed mental health professionals such as lay navigators. Tiered support for caregivers within stand-alone caregiver clinics may be one solution to challenges with reimbursement, staffing, and referral. Caregivers at low risk or with low distress levels may be appropriately managed by nonlicensed personnel who are trained in providing existing materials, whereas caregivers with moderate or high distress levels require care from licensed personnel (e.g., licensed mental health counselors, nurse practitioners, clinical psychologists, and psychiatrists). Furthermore, caregiver psychosocial care providers may benefit from working within existing teams of cancer care providers at cancer treatment clinics, on inpatient service lines, in survivorship clinics, and within general palliative care.

Common Ethical Dilemmas

Ethical dilemmas may arise when the presence of a caregiver is used as a criterion for specific treatments: for example, at most treatment facilities, bone marrow transplantation requires a primary caregiver to be available around the clock for 100 days post-transplant. Providers who identify caregivers with distress or psychosocial issues are morally and ethically bound to address these issues even if it may lead to the person with cancer being ineligible for transplant, which is a common practice in developed countries. In cases where caregivers have significant distress, addressing these issues early may enable them to continue or resume their caregiving role. In addition, caregivers with significant distress may be a risk to the persons they care for because their ability to provide care can be impacted by their own mental health deterioration. An additional dilemma is that stand-alone caregiver clinics are not widely available.

Policies

Disparities exist in the resources that are necessary to provide effective services to mitigate the unmet needs of caregivers. It may cause differing degrees of caregiver unmet needs and health consequences across various subgroups. Generalizability of current knowledge to caregivers who reside in low- and middle-income countries or rural regions and who may have limited education and income is limited. Moreover, caregivers who are also from historically underrepresented races or ethnicities (e.g., Black, Indigenous, Asian, Hispanic) or sexual orientation and gender identity (e.g., LGBTQ+) and facing greater health disparities may require a higher level of psychosocial care and support. National organizations, such as the American Cancer Society (ACS CARES: https://www.cancer.org/support-programs-and-servi ces/acs-cares.htmlNa) and the National Alliance for Caregiving (Cancer Caregiving Collaborative: https://www.caregiving.org/cancer-caregiving-collaborative/), as well as international organizations such as International Psycho-Oncology Society (https://www.ipos-society.org/patients/resour ces), can be useful resources. These organizations also aim at policy and practice changes through evidence-based initiatives to implement systematic pathways to reduce the unmet needs of family caregivers, particularly those who are historically underserved, across patients' various illness trajectories and through bereavement.

Teams and Supervision

The role of caregivers in the healthcare system is often seen as an obligation and duty to the person with cancer. Ongoing challenges in professional responsibility over caregiver health and well-being exist due to a host of reasons ranging from staffing shortages and workload issues in cancer care and survivorship to unclear referral pathways and financing issues. Standardization of care for caregivers is needed, but, until then, the responsibility for caregiver psychosocial health lies with those cancer treatment providers, clinics, and hospitals who interact with caregivers throughout the cancer trajectory.

References

1. Kim Y, Ting A, Carver CS, et al. International collaboration for assessing unmet needs of cancer survivors and family caregivers: Lens of healthcare professionals. Psycho-Oncology. 2023;32(1):77–85. doi: 10.1002/pon.6051.

2. Geng HM, Chuang DM, Yang F, et al. Prevalence and determinants of depression in caregivers of cancer patients: A systematic review and meta-analysis. Medicine. 2018;97(39):e11863. doi: ARTN e1186310.1097/MD.0000000000011863.

3. Kim Y, Kashy DA, Spillers RL, Evans TV. Needs assessment of family caregivers of cancer survivors: Three cohorts comparison. Psycho-Oncology. 2010;19(6):573–582. doi: 10.1002/pon.1597.

4. Vroom VH. Some personality determinants of the effects of participation. J Abnorm Soc Psych. 1959;59(3):322–327. doi: 10.1037/h0049057.

5. Grassi L, Fujisawa D, Odyio P, et al. Disparities in psychosocial cancer care: A report from the International Federation of Psycho-oncology Societies. Psycho-Oncology. 2016;25(10):1127–1136. doi: 10.1002/pon.4228.

6. Travado L, Breitbart W, Grassi L, et al. 2015 President's Plenary International Psycho-oncology Society: Psychosocial care as a human rights issue-challenges and opportunities. Psycho-Oncology. 2017;26(4):563–569. doi: 10.1002/pon.4209.

7. Kim Y, Carver CS, Ting A, Cannady RS. Passages of cancer caregivers' unmet needs across 8 years. Cancer-Am Cancer Soc. 2020. doi: 10.1002/cncr.33053.

8. American Psychiatric Association. Diagnostic and Statistical Manual of Mental Disorders (5th ed.). American Psychiatric Association; 2023.

9. Webb K, Sharpe L, Butow P, et al. Caregiver fear of cancer recurrence: A systematic review and meta-analysis of quantitative studies. Psycho-Oncology. 2023;32(8):1173–1191. doi: 10.1002/pon.6176.

10. Thomas TH CG, Tan KR, et al. Integrating family caregivers into cancer care: Implementation of evidence-based caregiver protocols Into gynecologic oncology practice. JCO Oncology Practice. 2024. doi: 10.1200/OP.24.00383.

11. Applebaum AJ, Schofield E, Kastrinos A, et al. A randomized controlled trial of a distress screening, consultation, and targeted referral system for family caregivers in oncologic care. Psycho-Oncology. 2024;33(2):e6301. doi: ARTN e630110.1002/pon.6301.

12. Sadigh G, Switchenko J, Weaver KE, et al. Correlates of financial toxicity in adult cancer patients and their informal caregivers. Support Care Cancer. 2022;30(1):217–225. doi: 10.1007/s00520-021-06424-1.

13. Given CW, Given B, Stommel M, Collins C, King S, Franklin S. The caregiver reaction assessment (CRA) for caregivers to persons with chronic physical and mental impairments. Res Nurs Health. 1992;15(4):271–283. doi: 10.1002/nur.4770150406.

14. Mutsaers B, Rutkowski N, Jones G, Lamarche J, Lebel S. Assessing and managing patient fear of cancer recurrence. Can Fam Physician. 2020;66(9):672–673.

15. Michopoulos I, Douzenis A, Kalkavoura C, et al. Hospital Anxiety and Depression Scale (HADS): Validation in a Greek general hospital sample. Ann Gen Psychiatry. 2008;7:4. doi: 10.1186/1744-859X-7-4.

16. Kroenke K, Spitzer RL, Williams JB. The PHQ-9: Validity of a brief depression severity measure. J Gen Intern Med. 2001;16(9):606–613. doi: 10.1046/j.1525-1497.2001.016009606.x.

17. Sancho-Domingo C, Carballo JL, Coloma-Carmona A, Buysse DJ. Brief version of the Pittsburgh Sleep Quality Index (B-PSQI) and measurement invariance across gender and age in a population-based sample. Psychol Assess. 2021;33(2):111–121. doi: 10.1037/pas0000959.

18. Faschingbauer T. The Texas Inventory of Grief – Revised. Honeycomb Publishing; 1981.

19. American Psychiatric Association. Clinical practice guidelines. 2025. https://www.psychiatry.org/psychiatrists/practice/clinical-practice-guidelines

20. Kusi G, Atenafu EG, Boamah Mensah AB, et al. The effectiveness of psychoeducational interventions on caregiver-oriented outcomes in caregivers of adult cancer patients: A systematic review and meta-analysis. Psycho-Oncology. 2023;32(2):189–202. doi: 10.1002/pon.6050.

21. Kim M, Tan KR, Coombs LA. Efficacy of web-based interventions on depression and anxiety in cancer caregivers: A systematic review and meta-analysis. Psycho-Oncology 2024;33(7):e9301. https://doi.org/10.1002/pon.9301

22. Chow R, Mathews JJ, Cheng EY, et al. Interventions to improve outcomes for caregivers of patients with advanced cancer: A meta-analysis. J Natl Cancer Instit. 2023;115(8):896–908. https://doi.org/10.1093/jnci/djad075

23. Reblin M, Ketcher D, McCormick R, et al. A randomized wait-list controlled trial of a social support intervention for caregivers of patients with primary malignant brain tumor. Bmc Health Serv Res. 2021;21(1):360. doi: 10.1186/s12913-021-06372-w.

24. Otto AK, Ketcher D, Reblin M, Terrill AL. Positive psychology approaches to interventions for cancer dyads: A scoping review. Int J Env Res Pub Health. 2022;19(20):13561. doi: 10.3390/jerph192013561.

25. Han AR, Yuen HK, Jenkins J, Lee HY. Acceptance and Commitment Therapy (ACT) guided online for distressed caregivers of persons living with dementia. Clin Gerontologist. 2022;45(4):927–938. doi: 10.1080/07317115.2021.1908475.

26. Ye F, Lee JJ, Xue D, Yu DS. Acceptance and commitment therapy among informal caregivers of people with chronic health conditions: A systematic review and meta-analysis. JAMA Netw Open. 2023;6(12):e2346216. doi: 10.1001/jamanetworkopen.2023.46216.

27. Kohle N, Drossaert CHC, Ten Klooster PM, et al. Web-based self-help intervention for partners of cancer patients based on acceptance and commitment therapy and self-compassion training: A randomized controlled trial with automated versus personal feedback. Support Care Cancer. 2021;29(9):5115–5125. doi: 10.1007/s00520-021-06051-w.

28. Applebaum AJ, Panjwani AA, Buda K, et al. Emotion regulation therapy for cancer caregivers: An open trial of a mechanism-targeted approach to addressing caregiver distress. Transl Behav Med. 2020;10(2):413–422. doi: 10.1093/tbm/iby104.

29. Applebaum AJ, Baser RE, Roberts KE, et al. Meaning-centered psychotherapy for cancer caregivers: A pilot trial among caregivers of patients with glioblastoma multiforme. Transl Behav Med. 2022;12(8):841–852. doi: 10.1093/tbm/ibac043.

30. Spicer L. Eye Movement Desensitisation and Reprocessing (EMDR) therapy for prolonged grief: Theory, research, and practice. Front Psychiatry. 2024;15:1357390. doi: 10.3389/fpsyt.2024.1357390.

Chapter 7

Return to Work

Saskia F. A. Duijts, Margaret I. Fitch, and
Susanne Oksbjerg Dalton

Learning Objectives

After reading this chapter, the clinician will be able to:

1. Identify and address barriers that cancer patients and survivors face when returning to and maintaining work during or after treatment.
2. Identify patients at risk for not returning to work and financial toxicity.
3. Apply or refer to personalized support programs and strategies, ensuring sustainable work retention for cancer patients and survivors.

Background Evidence

Approximately half of all patients with cancer receive their diagnosis during their working years.[1] This requires a person who is entering a period of high medical uncertainty and burden to make arrangements regarding work, such as using sick leave, communicating the diagnosis to colleagues, or retaining tasks at work in close consultation with their employer. Even for those without traditional employment, such as self-employed individuals or those receiving social benefits, work is a topic that needs attention because governmental or corporate offices may need to be informed of the person's disability.[2,3] Thus, the question "Do you need support regarding work?" is both justified and relevant. This is further emphasized by rising survival rates that enable more patients with cancer to return to work post-treatment or continue working during treatment.[1,4]

Addressing work-related concerns in clinical practice is vital due to the growing number of cancer patients and survivors and the meaning of work in general. Beyond financial security, work provides emotional well-being and a feeling of control during a time of physical and psychological challenges. It can help maintain a sense of normalcy, provide social interactions, and offer a structured environment that can serve as a positive distraction from the stress associated with illness and treatment. Many people derive a significant portion of their identity and self-worth from their professional role.[5]

Cancer and its treatments can significantly compromise the capacity to work. Not only the symptoms from the cancer itself, but also the acute side effects and long-term effects of cancer treatment may have an impact on the ability to meet job requirements. Unemployment is an example of an adverse work outcome, and it is 40% higher among cancer survivors than in people who have never been diagnosed with cancer.[6] Increased risk of receiving disability benefits was found in cancer survivors compared to the general population.[2,7] Such adverse outcomes are associated with a higher risk of *financial toxicity* (i.e., the financial burden faced by cancer patients and survivors).[8] Workplace stigma, discrimination, and lack of support from coworkers and employers further compound these challenges.

Numerous factors influence cancer survivors' ability to return to work: older age, female gender, lower educational level, diagnosis- and treatment-related factors (e.g., type of cancer, advanced stage, extensive treatment, comorbidities), and high levels of fatigue, depression, and cognitive problems. Workplace factors, such as job-related stress, lack of support, and physically demanding roles, further diminish return-to-work prospects. Moreover, sociolegal systems and cultural contexts influence the ability to reintegrate and show significant variability across countries.[9–11]

Given the financial and social challenges faced by working-age cancer patients and survivors, supporting their return to and retention of work during or after treatment is important. Healthcare professionals can play a pivotal role by addressing work-related issues early in the illness trajectory, potentially mitigating long-term adverse outcomes including financial hardship.

Presenting Problems

Up to one-third of cancer survivors with acute treatment-related symptoms or long-term treatment effects are unable to return to work, and more than half of survivors are not able to work as they had before their diagnosis; these individuals will require flexible and accommodated work arrangements.

Key Symptoms and Signs

The symptoms that may influence the ability to perform work-related activities and meet job requirements could be physical, cognitive, emotional, or psychological and may have an impact during primary cancer treatment as well as after treatment has finished (see Table 7.1).

- *Physical symptoms.* Everyone is different when it comes to experiencing the impact of physical symptoms and whether these impact directly on one's ability to fulfill job requirements. Symptoms such as fatigue can influence readiness and motivation to work, while changes in bowel habits can cause difficulties depending on the work environment and how easy it is to access washroom facilities. It is important that cancer survivors and their healthcare professionals review the expected acute side effects and long-term treatment effects together and determine how these will influence specific job expectations and requirements.

- *Cognitive symptoms.* Many cancer survivors report changes in their cognitive abilities, especially those who have received chemotherapy or have received radiation to the head. Survivors report various levels of

Table 7.1 Cancer symptoms which may affect work ability

Physical		Cognitive	Emotional and psychological
Fatigue, deconditioning	Changes in skin and nails	Concentration/ ability to focus	Changes in mood/ emotional reactions
Sleep disturbances	Infections	Ability to multi-task	Feelings of stigma and discrimination
Challenges in eating/nutrition	Difficulty communicating	Harder to learn new information	Feelings of stress and anxiety
Nerve damage, paresthesia, neuropathy	Changes in physical appearance, body image, disfigurement	Difficulty recalling previously learned information or finding words while speaking or writing	Lack of motivation/ readiness/feelings of uncertainty
Changes in bowel and bladder function	Mobility impairments	Difficulty making decisions	Sense of poor coping, loss of confidence or morale
Hot flashes	Hearing impairment		
Breathing difficulties	Visual impairment		
Nausea and vomiting	Lymphedema		
Pain	Seizures		
Bleeding problems			

difficulty concentrating and remembering details, learning new information, and solving problems. They can have trouble organizing work, answering questions quickly, shifting from one task to another, and recalling instructions. For most individuals, these cognitive symptoms will disappear over time, yet mild cognitive symptoms have been found to be present up to 20 years after treatment completion.

- *Emotional and psychological symptoms.* Most individuals will have an emotional response to receiving a cancer diagnosis and undergoing treatment. Coping with the inability to work and the potential increased financial burden is likely to add to present feelings of stress and anxiety. Some may feel relief at not having to work, while others will be worried about financial repercussions and fearful of job insecurity. The burden of not working can have a profound influence on a person's identity. Individuals with a strong work identity often have higher job satisfaction and productivity. This identity can be threatened if a person is not working or experiences job loss.

Returning to work following treatment may be a time of uncertainty and worry, but it also can bring about a sense of life returning to normal. For some, it may also lead to questions about the nature of the job and whether the person wishes to continue in their present position. Once back at work, individuals could experience fears of not being able to perform, frustration with the job requirements, or sadness at their employer's reactions.

Discrimination and stigmatization still occur in some work settings when individuals diagnosed with cancer continue or return to work.

The specific impact of symptoms and long-term effects on work will vary from individual to individual based on several factors. Some of these factors are modifiable, while others are not. These factors include:

- The type and prognosis of the cancer
- The type and intensity of treatment
- The nature, intensity, and requirements of the job (i.e., a job in building construction or waiting tables in a restaurant will be different from a position in teaching or accountancy)
- Workplace support
- Availability of personal finances
- Personality and personal values relating to work
- Access to healthcare
- The social security system

Misperceptions often exist on the part of coworkers and employers about cancer, cancer recurrence, and the survivor's ability to work and be productive. Survivors report lack of flexibility offered in work schedules, lack of graduated re-entry to work, lack of job opportunities, and difficulty communicating with employers about their needs for accommodation. These issues may raise concerns on the part of cancer survivors about whether they should inform their employer or their coworkers about their cancer diagnosis; the choice to disclose a diagnosis of cancer, or any illness, always rests with the patient.

It is crucial for healthcare professionals to understand the financial and social consequences of not working. Cancer patients and survivors need access to clear, easy-to-understand information on existing policies and legislation on return to work and job retention, as well as on available support programs and social security coverage.[12]

Caregivers

Similar issues exist for family caregivers of individuals with cancer in terms of their work-related activity. Caregivers can be involved in providing a range of care activities (e.g., emotional/informational support, physical care, financial manager, advocate) that can change during the course of treatment. Often, they will require periods of time away from their own work or accommodated work arrangements. Caregivers have also reported difficulties in finding support from employers regarding necessary arrangements and receiving unhelpful feedback from coworkers. Healthcare providers and employers must understand that the workplace is often a welcome opportunity for caregivers to focus on matters other than cancer and caregiving responsibilities.

Investigations for Key Differential Diagnoses

The issue of staying at work or returning to work is relevant for working-age patients and survivors throughout their disease trajectory (e.g., at time of diagnosis, during treatment, at times of progression or relapse, and after treatment completion).[13] At each of these timepoints it may be prudent to review and revise decisions concerning employment for the patient, survivor, and caregivers. It is relevant to establish a dialogue about work and to start this dialogue early after diagnosis or at the beginning of the treatment trajectory. This early dialogue is important because not discussing work may negatively affect patients' ability to return to work and impact related issues such as financial security[14] (see Boxes 7.1 and 7.2).

It is important to assess if the individual will be physically, cognitively, emotionally, and psychologically able to continue work or return to work; to offer counsel regarding which symptoms may be expected and what their impact will be on staying at work or returning to work; and to discuss what options the patient may have regarding sick leave and rehabilitation.[11] Several validated measurement tools are available for differential work-related issues (see Appendix A, "Measurement Tools for Differential Work-Related Issues"). Furthermore, if the patient will be permanently too sick to return to work, this should be discussed and documented during the process of obtaining disability benefits, pension (full or partial), or early retirement.

Box 7.1 Patients at Risk for Not Returning (Fully) to Work

- Young patients without a secure footing in the jobs market
- Older patients approaching retirement age
- Patients with a lower educational level
- Patients who had a loose affiliation with jobs market prior to cancer (e.g., those receiving unemployment or social benefits)
- Patients who hold unskilled and/or physically demanding jobs
- Patients with comorbidity that may affect their work ability
- Patients with ethnic minority backgrounds
- Patients with a large symptom burden affecting work ability
- Patients with specific cancer types (e.g., rare cancers)

Box 7.2 Risk Factors for Financial Toxicity

- Being female
- Extremes of age (younger, older)
- Race/ethnic minorities
- Lower (household) annual income
- Lower financial reserves/resources
- Sole provider
- Loss of income during treatment
- No or inadequate healthcare insurance (in countries where this is relevant)
- Less security in employment status/self-employment
- Low financial acumen
- Selected household structures: large families, social isolation

Considering the resources available, the healthcare professional should discuss with the cancer survivor about the need for a referral to a social worker, specialized occupational physician, or occupational rehabilitation unit for advice and/or support. The individual may wish to have support regarding, for example, communicating with their employer when asking for reduced hours due to lessened work ability during treatment, or, when reintegrating into work life after treatment is finalized, when some more permanent reasonable changes to work tasks or hours may be relevant.

For some patients and survivors not working may have greater consequences than for others. For example, in the case of being a sole provider, the paradox of not feeling able to work but needing the income will be of great concern. For many patients, worrying about work is not a priority when they are in the middle of diagnosis and treatment initiation, and they may not really want to talk about work when a healthcare professional first raises the issue. However, studies have shown that when the issue of work is raised, patients are reassured that the healthcare professional knows this may become an issue. It is important to offer the patient an opportunity to raise work-related concerns at a later time.

As with many important issues in cancer survivors' life and health, healthcare professionals should proactively ask about work-related issues throughout their contacts with patients because work ability often changes with time according to symptoms, prognosis, and the patient's and family's ability to cope.

Clinical Management

A range of psycho-educational, vocational, physical, and multicomponent programs and strategies have been developed to support cancer survivors' return to work or continuation of work after a return. Physical exercise or rehabilitation programs developed to improve cancer survivors' physical functioning and counteract negative physical consequences of cancer and its treatment have shown some positive impact on returning to and staying at work.[1]

Multicomponent programs, in which elements of psycho-educational, vocational, and/or physical/exercise strategies are combined to ameliorate adverse work outcomes, seem to be most promising. Specifically, more success is seen when all important stakeholders (e.g., patients, family, employers, occupational rehabilitation experts) are involved.[15]

Although evidence from research studies is sparse, it is important that healthcare professionals *know*, *ask*, and *do*. The timing of delivery and the type and intensity of supportive interventions and care should be taken into account.

What Healthcare Professionals Need to Know, Ask, and Do per Disease Phase

Diagnostic Phase

- The patient's physical, emotional, and social well-being should be carefully considered in relation to the topic of work.

- When it concerns work-related issues and meeting a patient's need for early information provision, the first point of contact in the hospital should be a nurse navigator, social worker, or occupational therapist. These healthcare professionals should ask about details of current work, if there is a need for sick leave or reduced working hours, or if an existing sick leave should be prolonged.
- Focus on the needs of the patient and raise awareness of the trajectory for return to work, related laws and regulations, and the potential financial impact of time off or reduced hours (see Box 7.2).
  - Refer the patient to "cancer-and-work" experts in- or outside the hospital if additional advice or information is required.
- Encourage patients to initiate and maintain contact with their occupational physician, direct work supervisor, and colleagues, and ask questions such as: "What support do you have from your employer?" or "Are there any legal or financial aspects you are worried about?"
- Informal contact with colleagues and employers can be helpful for emotional processing.
- Explore pre-treatment symptoms that may affect work ability in cases where a patient wishes to continue work.

Treatment Phase

- When a patient expresses a wish to continue working during treatment, the treatment plan and potential (long-term or late) physical and mental effects (such as fatigue, pain, cognitive changes, anxiety) should be considered in line with the patient's job demands and the degree of flexibility and available accommodations at work.
  - Physical/exercise rehabilitation programs during treatment have been found to be effective on earlier return to work and when patient's wish to work more hours per week.[15]
- Ask: "Do you have concerns about managing work and treatment?" or "Do you have concerns about affording medications, travel to appointments, or other treatment-related expenses?" to identify potential (financial) challenges the patient foresees in balancing work with ongoing treatment.
- Explore the patient's expectations regarding work and whether the patient's social network (e.g., partner or family members) supports the choice to continue work.
- A social worker or psychologist can be involved to ensure the patient has a comprehensive support system in place. If the patient's employer and colleagues consider it challenging when the patient continues to work during treatment, the patient can be referred to occupational support as (additional) difficulties at work may arise.
- Be aware that cancer treatment can lead to significant out-of-pocket costs, loss of income, and financial stress, which can negatively impact patients' mental health and adherence to treatment.
- Familiarize yourself to some extent with the social security system, disability benefits, and financial aid programs in your country and/or know who to refer patients to.

- Modify the "work during treatment" plan if acute symptoms make work more challenging.

Post-Treatment Phase

- Questions about work may emerge when patients start to physically recover from cancer and its treatment, such as "Do I want to, need to, or have to return to work?" and "Am I able to, and what do I need to return to work?"
- The potential for long-term or late effects of cancer and the treatment received should be discussed in the context of work ability, such as cognitive impairment, hormonal changes, or increased susceptibility to infections.
- Referral to adequate rehabilitation programs should be based on symptoms and needs as well as on the wishes of the patient.
  - Cognitive strategy programs for occupationally active cancer survivors who experience cognitive symptoms at work have been found to be effective when it concerns attaining personal work goals.[16]
- Information could be provided by, for example, a reintegration consultant or a (clinical) occupational physician.
- Communication and coordination between healthcare providers (including general practitioners, social workers, and occupational physicians) is important during this phase.

Advanced Care Phase

- Leaving the workforce permanently can be an emotionally challenging transition for which support can and should be provided. Questions could include, "Should work disability be assessed or (early) disability pension be obtained?"
- Navigating financial support systems can be complex, and timely advice about or referral to support regarding disability claims, insurance, and income replacement is crucial.
- For patients whose symptoms become more manageable, returning to work—either part-time or in a different capacity—might be an option. A palliative care team may be involved to provide patients with guidance on realistic goals regarding their work and well-being.
  - Patients can be confronted with social discomfort when they do not seem to fulfill the expectations of their environment regarding being incurably ill.[17]

Case Study

Maria, a 56-year-old administrative assistant, was diagnosed with breast cancer a year ago. After completing her treatment, she was eager to return to work but faced significant challenges. Despite her physical recovery, fatigue, limited mobility in her right arm after surgery, and lingering emotional distress often left her feeling unprepared for a full workload. Maria's employer, a small company, showed little understanding of her situation. Her requests for flexible hours or remote work were denied, with her manager insisting she either resume her full duties or take unpaid leave. Feeling unsupported, Maria became increasingly anxious. The lack of workplace accommodation and her fear of job loss began to weigh heavily on her, exacerbating her emotional and physical struggles. Financially, the situation became dire. Maria's reduced income strained the household, and she worried about covering future medical costs.

Maria's husband Carlos, a 58-year-old construction worker, tried his best to support Maria emotionally and financially. He took on additional hours at his job to cover their expenses, but the physical toll left him exhausted. Watching Maria struggle to regain her confidence and independence was heartbreaking. He felt powerless to help her navigate the complexities of returning to work or addressing the financial strain.

Maria's oncologist noticed her heightened anxiety during a routine follow-up and referred her to a social worker. The social worker helped Maria access vocational rehabilitation services, connecting her with a career counselor who advocated for workplace accommodations. A consultation with a physical therapist addressed Maria's mobility issues, while a psychologist provided coping strategies for her emotional well-being. To prevent financial hardship, Maria's healthcare team recommended speaking with a financial counselor, who assisted in exploring government disability benefits and support programs for cancer survivors. They also facilitated a meeting between Maria, her employer, and a labor expert to mediate reasonable adjustments, such as gradual workload increases.

With professional support, Maria gradually reintegrated into her job and her employer adopted a more flexible stance. This improved her mental health, eased her financial strain, and restored her sense of purpose. Carlos, relieved to see progress, felt empowered to focus on his own well-being, and their family regained stability.

This case illustrates that healthcare professionals in oncology should know about available psychosocial support and vocational interventions so that they can counsel and refer for relevant supportive care to those patients struggling with return to work.

Professional Issues and Service Implementation

Recording and Communicating

There is no global consensus on whether dealing with work-related impacts from cancer and cancer treatment should be the purview of cancer specialists. As a result, healthcare professionals within the cancer setting may not consider work-related concerns as part of an individual's plan of care, believing instead that this topic is the responsibility of community-based services, not hospital or cancer center staff. In other situations, healthcare professionals within the cancer setting may be expected only to have initial conversations to identify the need for sick leave notices. To equip patients for what they may expect in terms of return to work requires healthcare professionals to understand work-related issues and their potential impacts as well as the available rehabilitation programs, late-effects services, and/or job strategies relevant to cancer survivors. Both specialists in cancer centers as well as practitioners in the primary care setting should have conversations with patients or survivors about the need to consult occupational experts if necessary.

Referrals

Some cancer programs will have staff members who can provide in-depth information and support regarding work-related issues, while others may develop referral pathways for necessary resolution. Medical specialists and nurses are often the first to recognize when a referral is needed to identify challenges that may hinder a patient's return to work (e.g., to social workers, financial navigators, occupational therapists, specialized or general rehabilitation services, pain specialists) based on work-related concerns expressed by the patient.

Legal Responsibilities

There are various laws and policies in existence to protect cancer survivors and/or caregivers in terms of work-related issues. These regulations can cover insurance, contracts, workers compensation, and employment equity. However, there is wide variation from jurisdiction to jurisdiction regarding the existence of these laws and whether cancer or its consequences to health is considered a disability. For the most part, individuals diagnosed with cancer are entitled to reasonable accommodation in their workplace, which includes flexible working hours, ability to work at home, time off for appointments, and change in duties that can no longer be performed. Such accommodation may allow individuals to continue to perform productively in their employment and thus offset financial toxicity. Moreover, governments ought to implement proactive return-to-work programs for cancer patients and survivors and provide relevant sick leave benefits.

Common Ethical Dilemmas

When making decisions related to work or in dealing with discrimination following their diagnosis, cancer survivors must know their rights concerning work laws, regulations, and policies. It is important that individuals know what rights they have or what arrangements regarding time off work they are entitled to receive. A specific question cancer patients or survivors must consider is the issue of disclosing their diagnosis. Sharing information about their cancer diagnosis is the right of the individual. Whether or not an individual tells an employer and/or coworkers about their diagnosis is the person's own decision. This applies whether the person is currently employed or seeking a job after the diagnosis.

Unfortunately, there are still situations where cancer survivors are experiencing discrimination, such as being asked to quit working because of cancer or being reassigned to a job with less demanding duties or less pay without the cancer survivor's permission. In such cases, healthcare professionals may support patients and survivors by providing documentation about symptoms related to cancer and its treatment.

Teams and Supervision

Multidisciplinary teams supporting patients and survivors throughout treatment and follow-up typically include medical cancer specialists, nurses, and allied health professionals. Ideally, to support return to work, such teams should also include occupational physicians and occupational therapists, and, preferably, these teams should operate across hospital-based cancer centers, rehabilitation clinics, and community healthcare settings, thus requiring strong administrative coordination to ensure integrated care. Supervision for staff managing return-to-work issues should be provided by senior specialists within their respective disciplines.

References

1. Ferlay J, Colombet M, Soerjomataram I, Dyba T, Randi G, Bettio M, et al. Cancer incidence and mortality patterns in Europe: Estimates for 40 countries and 25 major cancers in 2018. Eur J Cancer 2018;103:356–387.

2. Paalman CH, van Leeuwen FE, Aaronson NK, et al. Employment and social benefits up to 10 years after breast cancer diagnosis: A population-based study. Br J Cancer. 2016;114(1):81–87.

3. Van Hoof E. *How Do Self-Employed Cancer Patients Experience Return-to-Work/Life after Treatment? Report for the Belgian Foundation Against Cancer.* Belgian Foundation against Cancer; 2015.

4. American Cancer Society. Cancer facts & figures. 2024. https://www.cancer.org/cancer/survivorship/be-healthy-after-treatment/returning-to-work-after-cancer-treatment.html.

5. Butow P, Laidsaar-Powell R, Konings S, Lim CYS, Koczwara B. Return to work after a cancer diagnosis: A meta-review of reviews and a meta-synthesis of recent qualitative studies. J Cancer Surviv. 2020;14(2):114–134.

6. de Boer AGEM, Taskila T, Ojajärvi A, van Dijk FJ, Verbeek JH. Cancer survivors and unemployment: A meta-analysis and metaregression. JAMA. 2009;301:753–762.

7. Hauglann BK, Saltytė Benth J, Fosså SD, Tveit KM, Dahl AA. A controlled cohort study of sickness absence and disability pension in colorectal cancer survivors. Acta Oncol. 2014;53(6):735–743.

8. Zafar SY. Financial toxicity of cancer care: It's time to intervene, JNCI. 2016;108:5.

9. Islam T, Dahlui M, Majid HA, Nahar AM, Mohd Taib NA, Su TT; MyBCC study group. Factors associated with return to work of breast cancer survivors: A systematic review. BMC Public Health. 2014;14:S8.

10. Wolvers MDJ, Leensen MCJ, Groeneveld IF, Frings-Dresen MHW, De Boer AGEM. Predictors for earlier return to work of cancer patients. J Cancer Surviv. 2018;12:169–177.

11. de Boer AGEM, de Wind A, Coenen P, et al. Cancer survivors and adverse work outcomes: Associated factors and supportive interventions. Br Med Bull. 2023;145(1):60–71.

12. European Commission: European Health and Digital Executive Agency; Buckingham S, Colonnese F, Broughton A. Study on job retention and return to work for cancer patients and survivors: Final study report. Publications Office of the European Union; 2024.

13. Duijts SFA. Management of work through the seasons of cancer survivorship. Curr Opin Support Palliat Care. 2018;12(1):80–85.

14. Zegers AD, Coenen P, van Belzen M, et al. Cancer survivors' experiences with conversations about work-related issues in the hospital setting. Psycho-Oncology. 2021;30(1):27–34.

15. de Boer AGEM, Tamminga SJ, Boschman JS, Hoving JL. Non-medical interventions to enhance return to work for people with cancer. Cochrane Database Syst Rev. 2024;3(3):CD007569.

16. Klaver KM, Duijts SFA, Geusgens CAV, et al. Internet-based cognitive rehabilitation for working cancer survivors: Results of a multicenter randomized controlled trial. JNCI Cancer Spectr. 2024;8(1):pkad110.

17. Beerda DCE, Zegers AD, van Andel ES, et al. Experiences and perspectives of patients with advanced cancer regarding work resumption and work retention: A qualitative interview study. Support Care Cancer. 2022;30(12):9713–9721.

Further Reading and Resources

Brink E, Pilegaard MS, Bonnesen TG, Nielsen CV, Pedersen P. Employment status in cancer patients the first five years after diagnosis-a register-based study. J Cancer Surviv. 2024;19(5):1598–1610. doi:10.1007/s11764-024-01576-5.

This paper highlights the long-term impact cancer can have on employment and emphasizes the need for increasing awareness of challenges regarding work-life after cancer.

Fitch MI, Nicoll I. Returning to work after cancer: Survivors', caregivers', and employers' perspectives. Psycho-Oncology. 2019;28(4):792–798.

This paper describes that multiple strategies from a range of stakeholders are needed to achieve success regarding returning to work after cancer: in-depth understanding of the work-related issues, consideration of work accommodation, adequate communication and education, resources, and financial support.

Lamore K, Dubois T, Rothe U, Leonardi M, et al. Return to work interventions for cancer survivors: A systematic review and a methodological critique. Int J Environ Res Public Health. 2019;16(8):1343.

This review underscores the necessity for consensus on return-to-work definitions and assessment methods to enhance the effectiveness of future interventions.

Møller JK, la Cour K, Pilegaard MS, et al. Social vulnerability among cancer patients and changes in vulnerability during their trajectories: A longitudinal population-based study. Cancer Epidemiol. 2023;85:102401.

This paper describes the difficulty of identifying socially vulnerable cancer patients in the healthcare system and highlights how patients' status of social vulnerability can change as several social and health-related indicators are involved in this complex multifactorial concept.

Stapelfeldt CM, Klaver KM, Rosbjerg RS, et al. A systematic review of interventions to retain chronically ill occupationally active employees in work: Can findings be transferred to cancer survivors? Acta Oncol. 2019;58(5):548–565.

Insights from this review highlight the potential for adapting successful work retention strategies from other chronic illness contexts to support cancer survivors in maintaining employment.

Websites

https://www.macmillan.org.uk/cancer-information-and-support/impacts-of-cancer/work-and-cancer Offers practical guidance and resources on balancing cancer treatment with employment, including legal rights and workplace adjustments. https://www.cancerandwork.ca/ Provides tailored advice for cancer survivors and employers, covering return-to-work planning, workplace accommodations, and vocational rehabilitation.

Chapter 8

Spiritually Sensitive Care in Cancer Survivorship

Jayita Deodhar

Learning Objectives

After reading this chapter, the clinician will be able to:

1. Describe the importance of culturally sensitive spiritual care.
2. Understand the clinical presentations of cancer survivors with spiritual distress and be able to assess these concerns using appropriate methods.
3. Describe the differential diagnoses and principles of management for a basic understanding of cancer survivors' spiritual needs.
4. Understand different interventions appropriate to cancer survivors' spiritual concerns and prepare a referral pathway for specialist care as needed.
5. Understand professional and service development issues that will enhance spiritual care.

Background Evidence.

Spirituality is a broad term and concept that can be defined variously as "one's connection to the transcendent or the divine," "an individual's meaning and purpose," "the connections between oneself and others," and "the connection to one's deepest self."[1] In practice, the concept of "spiritual concerns" that encompass spiritual, existential, and religious matters may prove to be clinically more helpful. Spiritual concerns are commonly experienced in the context of a patient's cancer journey from diagnosis to survivorship, and they can cause significant distress that impacts quality of life.[1] Thus, identification of spiritual issues is essential to optimize quality of life.[2] Spirituality is considered distinct from religion, but some groups and individuals may find it difficult to completely separate the two terms. Religion has been defined as a set of values and practices adopted by a particular group in an organized manner.[3]

Spiritual distress among cancer survivors might be associated with the diagnosis of cancer, its effect on self-efficacy, and the need for information about dealing with their illness, including after treatment completion.[4] Spiritual distress is linked to anxiety levels, reduced hope, and lower psychological adjustment and satisfaction levels. The use of spiritual resources can lead to better adjustment with the illness experience, and has a positive effect on both mental and physical health-related quality of life. Survivors of cancer can use their spirituality in meaning-making, in trying to understand their illness, and, ultimately, in coping to make the transition to wellness.[3] Engaging in religious practices generally improves adjustment to cancer, providing a greater sense of meaning and purpose, improved self-care, and better support for family and caregivers. Interventions that address the spiritual concerns of survivors should be based on their needs.

In the context of cancer survivorship, common spiritual concerns include anger toward God, meaning-seeking, fears about death, questioning the higher power or God, or feelings of shame and isolation. Forgiveness is another common spiritual concern for cancer survivors.

Prevalence of Spiritual Concerns

In a Danish study of 6,640 cancer survivors,[5] spiritual concerns were reported by one-fifth of the participants.[5] These concerns were most frequently associated with guilt or existential angst and were more common in patients of a younger age, women, and those with depression, anxiety, and loss of hope. Cannon et al. studied the relationships among spirituality, worry, and healthcare utilization at baseline, 6, and 12 months in 551 cancer survivors with different malignancies[6] in an oncology clinic in the United States, reporting that 280 (51%) had high spirituality scores.[6] Those with high spirituality were less likely to have worries at 6 and 12 months, but those with high worry scores were more likely to use healthcare resources. However, the authors did not find any significant interactions between spirituality and worry affecting utilization of healthcare.

Spiritual concerns vary among different cultural populations of cancer survivors. Among African American breast cancer survivors, despite being strongly spiritual, they still felt a sense of isolation.[7] In a meta-analysis of 15 qualitative studies on women with breast cancer from different ethnic and cultural groups, one of five major themes identified spirituality as being important in coping.[3] In a qualitative study with 20 Samoan breast cancer survivors, participants with strong spiritual beliefs used meaning-making to cope with the challenges of cancer survivorship.[8] In a mixed-method study of young adult survivors of racial/ethnic minority populations (Hispanics, Blacks, Asians, and Pacific Islanders), Munoz et al. described common qualitative themes surrounding emotions, changes in viewpoints, and social network support.[9] Although participants of Asian and Pacific Islander origin scored highly on appreciation of life, overall spiritual well-being did not differ significantly on quantitative measures among the various ethnic groups in this study. Although spiritual concerns are described in cancer survivors, some authors have reported on their resilience, growth, and transformation, especially in survivors who have lived long with incurable cancers.

Spiritually Sensitive Care for Cancer Survivors

Attention to cultural traditions alongside religious beliefs is essential to delivering person-centered care. These traditions might include the levels of family

Box 8.1 Definition of Culturally Sensitive Spiritual Care

In culturally sensitive care, a clinician responds appropriately to the customs, beliefs, feelings, or circumstances of a group of people that share a common and distinctive racial, ethic, linguistic, religious, or cultural heritage.

Adapted from U.S. Department of Health and Human Services, Office of Minority Health. National standards for culturally and linguistically appropriate services in health care: executive summary[Internet]. Rockville (MD): Office of Minority Health;2001 [cited 2025 Jan1], 13p. Available from: http://www.omhrc.gov/assest/pdf/checked/executive/pdf.

involvement when communicating about an illness and its management, understanding any key lay or folk beliefs about the illness experience (e.g., beliefs about contagion that may limit social support in some cultures), communication barriers, and how clinicians need to respond to culturally and linguistically diverse (CALD) communities. Certain team members (e.g., from psycho-oncology and chaplaincy professions) must be part of the support service for survivors. For a definition of culturally sensitive spiritual care,[10] see Box 8.1

Understanding Suffering

Team members from psycho-oncology and chaplaincy can help the entire team in understanding spirituality, including its measurement and assessment, and thereby provide a framework for delivering culturally and spiritually sensitive care.[11] Concepts like hope, dignity, and forgiveness are valuable in providing spiritual care. Therefore, oncology professionals have a duty to understand a cancer survivor's spiritual history alongside their cultural background and address their needs accordingly.

Presenting Problems

Cancer survivors have spiritual needs and concerns that, if unaddressed, can impede life in survivorship. They may experience different emotions in the context of the aftermath of treatment completion, struggle to return to routine life and work, have anger toward God, or question their meaning and purpose in life. Some spiritual symptoms that survivors might present with include

- Anger at God
- Doubts and uncertainties
- Fear they are being punished for prior actions or choices
- Guilt
- Loss of purpose and meaning in life
- Questioning God
- Sadness
- Sense of isolation

People who are survivors of a life-limiting illness like cancer go though different emotions as they face multidimensional issues, including spiritual concerns. "Why me?" is a question that most people will have, a feeling of being thrown into chaos. They might feel that their concerns are not being understood, and they tend to feel isolated. Stigma related to cancer can add to this sense of isolation.

Investigations for Key Differential Diagnoses

Four dimensions of spiritual needs should be assessed as follows:
- *Religiosity*: Personal religious and spiritual beliefs belonging to a particular religious community and religious rituals.
- *Spiritual well-being*: One of the measures of quality of life that can be negatively impacted by spiritual distress.
- *Spiritual needs*: Concerns arising from one's own beliefs in a higher transcendental power and connectedness, along with meaning and purpose in life; these needs often are affected by serious illness.
- *Spiritual or religious coping*: Use of religious and spiritual resources according to belief systems to help cope with a serious illness.

These domains are an integral part of screening, history-taking, and assessment, which can then determine specific interventions and help the patient and team plan pathways for specialist spiritual care.[1] Clinicians can follow this same approach in different cultures and communities.

When assessing spirituality in survivors, it is essential to establish a good rapport to enable a comprehensive history-taking. Factors such as belief system or faith, spiritual/religious practices, hopes and worries, meaning and purpose in life, coping strategies, and sources of psychosocial and spiritual support are important to ask about. Studies have found that although clinicians can be uncomfortable broaching the topic of spirituality with patients with cancer, about 52–58% of cancer survivors expect their clinicians to discuss their spiritual needs and concerns.[4]

Screening and History-Taking

Key questions regarding spirituality include the importance of religiosity or spirituality, meaning and belief systems, effects on or challenges to their goals and decision-making, connection to others and nature, and self-concept. One can also ask if the person is at peace.[1] This single question, although most often used in palliative care, also may be useful to identify the person who is facing a spiritual crisis in survivorship and is need of prompt intervention.[11]

The National Comprehensive Cancer Center's Distress Thermometer (NCCN-DT) is an easy to use self-report tool that measures distress from 0 (no distress) to 10 (severe distress), along with an associated 39-item Problem List for identifying sources of distress.[12] *Spiritual distress is one of the items listed as a source of distress.* The NCCN-DT is reliable and valid, with translations available in many languages. A score of 4 and above might point to a need for mental health evaluation of the cancer survivor. A score of less than 4, although not indicative of distress, may lead to exploration of supportive care needs.

🔍 Key Point

Several tools have been used for spiritual history-taking. Puchalski[13] developed the FICA tool (see Box 8.2), and Anandarajah and Hight [14] developed the HOPE tool as an alternative assessment of spiritual well-being (see Box 8.3).

Box 8.2 FICA Spiritual Assessment Tool

F: What is your faith or belief?

- Do you consider yourself spiritual or religious?
- What things do you believe in that give meaning to your life?

I: Is it important in your life?

- What influence does it have on how you take care of yourself?
- How have your beliefs influenced your behavior during this illness?
- What role do your beliefs play in regaining your health?

C: Are you part of a spiritual or religious community?

- Is this of support to you and how?
- Is there a person or group of people you really love or who are really important to you?

A: How would you like me, your healthcare provider, to address these issues?

Source: Puchalski CM. The FICA spiritual history tool #274. J Palliat Med. 2014;17(1):105–106. doi: 10.1089/JPM.2013.9458

Box 8.3 HOPE Approach to Spiritual Assessment

H: Spiritual resources:

- What are your sources of hope and peace?

O: Organized religion:

- Are you a member of an organized religion?
- What religious practices are important to you?

P: Personal spirituality:

- Do you have spiritual beliefs separate from organized religion?
- What spiritual practices are most helpful to you?

E: Effects on care:

- Is there any conflict between your beliefs and the care you will be receiving?
- Do you hold beliefs or follow practices that you believe may affect your care?
- Do you wish to consult with a religious or spiritual leader when you are ill or making decisions about your healthcare?

Source: Anandarajah G, Hight E. Spirituality and medical practice: Using the HOPE questions as a practical tool for spiritual assessment. Am Fam Physician. 2001;63(1):81–88. doi: 10.1016/S1443-8461(01)80044-7

Box 8.4 SPIRIT Assessment Tool

S– Spiritual belief system: Do you have a spiritual belief system? Do you have a formal religious affiliation? Can you elaborate? Do you consider your spiritual life to be important?

P –Personal spirituality: Describe the religious ideas and practices that you embrace. Describe the ideas and behaviors you do not embrace or adhere to. In what ways does your spirituality/religion mean something to you?

I – Integration with a spiritual community: Do you belong to any religious or spiritual organizations or communities? How do you interact with this group/community? What significance does this group hold for you? What kinds of support and assistance does or may this group offer you in coping with health issues?

R – Ritualized practices and restrictions: What specific practices do you engage in as part of your religious and spiritual life? What lifestyle habits or behaviors does your religion promote, discourage, or outright prohibit? How closely have you adhered to these guidelines?

I – Implications for medical practice: Is there any aspect of medical treatment that your faith discourages or prohibits? How closely have you adhered to these guidelines? What components of your religion/spirituality do you want me to remember while I care for you?

T – Terminal events planning: Are there any areas of medical care that you would like to avoid or have withheld due to your religion/spirituality? Do you want religious or spiritual rites or rituals to be offered in the hospital or at home? Are there any religious or spiritual traditions you would like to arrange for at the time of death or after death? How will your faith and spirituality impact your decisions as we arrange for your medical care at the end of life?

Source: Nolan TS, Browning K, Vo JB, Meadows RJ, Paxton RJ. Assessing and managing spiritual distress in cancer survivorship. Am J Nurs. 2020;120(1):40. doi: 10.1097/01.NAJ.0000652032.51780.56

The SPIRIT assessment tool (see Box 8.4) includes components of an individual's spiritual belief, personal spirituality, presence of integration with community, rituals and practice, implications for organizing care, and planning for terminal events.[4]

Other Measures

Other measures that can be used in cancer survivors for both clinical and research purposes include:

- *Spiritual Well-Being Scale* is a valid 20-item scale with two subscales of existential and religious well-being; it is available in different languages.[15]
- *Functional Assessment of Chronic Illness Therapy – Spiritual Well-Being Scale (FACIT-Sp)* is a valid 12-item scale measuring dimensions of meaning or

peace and faith, mainly used in clinical trials and translated into multiple languages.[16]

- *Spirituality Index of Well-Being (SIWB)* is a 12-item measure divided into two subscales; it is unique in including a self-efficacy domain along with a life-scheme domain.[17]
- *Spiritual Distress Assessment Tool (SDAT)* is another unique measure that has five open-ended questions that allow for an exploration of a person's meaning, values, and identity.[18]

These assessment tools have been developed and researched in the Western world with mainly White populations and may not translate well across all cultures. It is essential that culturally appropriate rating scales be established specifically for survivors in non-Caucasian populations, as was done with a scale established by Gielen et al.[19] for palliative care patients in India.

Differential Diagnoses

The prevalence of depression, anxiety, and post-traumatic stress symptoms is 11%, 18–20%, and 10%, respectively, in cancer survivors in different age groups.[20] Hence it is important to consider the following differential diagnosis when cancer survivors present with spiritual distress (see Chapters 2 and 4 for more details):

- *Major depressive disorder*: Guilt or sadness are prominent among the presenting symptoms.
- *Anxiety disorders*: fear is prominent among symptoms.[21]
- *Mood disorder secondary to medical condition*: Can be caused by endocrine, autoimmune, neurological, or organ dysfunctions or medications or malignancies.
- *Demoralization*: A loss of meaning, purpose, and hope are prominent among presenting symptoms, with ineffective coping and a sense of failure potentially leading to suicidal thoughts and resulting in negative outcomes.[22] Demoralization is incorporated as a specific syndrome in the latest edition of the *International Classification of Diseases* (ICD-11).
- *Post-traumatic stress disorder*: Intrusive thoughts and traumatic images are prominent, along with avoidant coping.[21]

Clinical Management

Difficulties can emerge when individuals face fundamental aspects of human existence, such as mortality, inherent solitude, the responsibilities that accompany freedom, and the quest for life's meaning. *It is crucial to recognize that existential distress can exacerbate depression.* Addressing spiritual distress is a vital element in a comprehensive care plan for cancer survivors, but creating a categorical framework for diagnosing spiritual distress is difficult and a diagnostic structure to document spiritual distress is not available. Nevertheless, an oncology professional should try to elicit a patient's concerns regarding spiritual beliefs, distress, and their impact on functioning by exploring the patient's personal beliefs and conflicts or dissonance with those, a loss of meaning and purpose, doubts about God or a higher power, beliefs about community or healthcare professionals, a decline in faith and hope, feelings of guilt, and experiences of grief. Profound distress may arise from an inability to find meaning and purpose in life or from losing faith and connection to oneself, nature, or a higher power.

A "problem list" or "concerns list" using the FICA, HOPE or SPIRIT tools can be effective to both document and ensure adequate coverage of these issues by the multidisciplinary team. While the diagnosis may correspond with adjustment disorder, the language used is often better left within the spiritual framework of these tools. It is essential to select the appropriate intervention and tailor it to the needs of the patient as a person.

Spiritual and Existential Interventions

Evidence is building that spiritually and existentially oriented interventions enhance well-being.[23–25] Bernacchi et al., in their qualitative study of rural cancer survivors in United States, have suggested inclusion of spirituality in any intervention because it facilitates resilience.[26]

NCCN guidelines recommend identifying, assessing, and making a care pathway for spiritual distress in cancer survivors as part of distress assessment and management.[27] The team providing survivorship care needs to be aware of its responsibility to provide spiritually sensitive care in a cultural competent manner. Nolan and colleagues[4] identified the following essential issues:

- *Respecting the beliefs of cancer survivors and acknowledging and exploring their concerns* using nonjudgemental exploration of concerns and active listening in a safe space.
- *Enabling survivors to incorporate their spiritual and religious beliefs into their care plans* by empowering them to integrate their own practices to create a holistic mind–body-oriented program.
- *Organizing a support system to address survivors' spiritual concerns* through seeking and creating peer groups, both formal professional-led and informal, to help navigate their spirituality.

Meaning-Centered Interventions

Meaning-centered interventions combine didactic elements, in which the therapist introduces various concepts of meaning at the start of each session, with experiential activities that allow patients to delve into the sources of meaning in their own lives.[28,29] The therapist covers concepts related to the significance of life, discovery of meaning in human existence, and the ability to find meaning in life even amid suffering.

Acceptance and Commitment Therapy

Acceptance and commitment therapy (ACT) is a form of cognitive behavioral therapy, which aims to alter the role of troubling or distressing thoughts rather than modifying or adjusting them. In ACT, acceptance involves actively focusing on rather than avoiding negative thoughts, feelings, and emotions and being fully engaged with them in the present moment. It entails a readiness to endure unwanted experiences if they are integral to pursuing what is meaningful to the individual. The effectiveness of ACT for cancer survivors has been reported by Mathew et al. in a systematic review of 13 articles covering 537 cancer survivors. ACT significantly improved outcomes on measures of anxiety, depression, and fear of cancer recurrence.[30]

Complementary Therapies

Complementary medicine, also referred to as *integrative medicine*, can reduce discomfort and promote well-being and may help address spiritual concerns. These approaches include mind–body or mindfulness practices such as meditation and yoga, energy medicine, and arts-based expressive therapies. Jones et al. has noted the role of complementary and alternative medicine to address spiritual issues in cancer survivors.[31] Mind–body interventions are useful for the holistic health and well-being of cancer survivors.

Other Interventions to Address Spiritual Concerns in Cancer Survivors

Authors have described different types of spirituality-related interventions for cancer survivors. Bastian et al. recommended *peer-led support groups* with an emphasis on sharing of personal culture and spirituality in their study of Native American survivors of cancers.[32] Singh-Carlson et al. studied breast cancer survivors of South Asian ethnicity in a qualitative study and noted that these women[33] described themes of their faith, "inner strength," and belief in karma impacting their experiences in moving on with their lives post-treatment. Bastian et al. have noted that survivors of certain ethnicities value the balance between resources based on modern medicine and the emphasis of their traditional medicine on spirituality and culture.[32]

Care Available in the Community

Cultural and regional differences exist among high-, middle-, and low-income countries and these restrict the generalizability of spiritual assessment tools and intervention measures for spiritual care. There is also a dearth of community-based studies on the spiritual care of, and interventions with, cancer survivors.

Case Study

Ms. R, an unmarried 32-year-old woman, was diagnosed with breast cancer at the age of 27 and underwent surgery followed by chemotherapy. At the time of diagnosis she was working in a clerical position in a private-sector company and lived with her mother, an elder brother, and an elder disabled sister. She had another elder sister who was married and lived nearby.

Ms. R was referred to the psycho-oncology department in the cancer hospital where she was getting her treatment because she had some pre-existing anxiety symptoms and apprehensions regarding treatment. The psycho-oncology team supported her and advised anxiety management techniques of relaxation and mindfulness, which she adhered to. She followed-up for her appointments regularly.

On spiritual assessment during her initial assessment, she said that she had faith in God and though she did not take part in any spiritual community, she had her own rituals that she practiced, like praying. She did not express having any unmet spiritual needs. She described her spirituality as "deepened" by her suffering and identified hope, purpose, and meaning in life as central to her healing.

During Ms. R's initial course of cancer treatment, most unfortunately, she had multiple losses. Her elder disabled sister, elder brother, and mother died within the span of a few months. These losses occurred amid the physical and emotional burden of cancer therapy. Superimposed on her profound grief, she faced home-lessness as her elder sister tried to oust her from her paternal home. Despite these adverse events, Ms. R continued her cancer treatment and followed-up with her clinic appointments.

During her treatment and follow-up, she depended on her psycho-oncology team for emotional and psychosocial support. Despite adversities, she continued to have faith in God and maintained her connection and therapeutic relationship with the psycho-oncology team. She said that this connection increased her resil-ience and gave her meaning in life.

The spiritual issues identified in this case study are the patient's strong sense of faith, meaning-making in her suffering and losses, processing of her grief related to multiple deaths in the family, and her strengths of hope and desire for connection. Using the FICA assessment approach, we can see that the pa-tient had faith, believed that spirituality was important, did not belong to any particular community, and was able to use her own coping along with support from the psycho-oncology team.

A spiritual care management plan for this patient should include support from the psycho-oncology team through meaning-making interventions, continuing assessment and monitoring for spiritual distress, referral to a spir-itual counselor if required, and a survivorship care plan incorporating spiritu-ality in the comprehensive management program for her smooth transition to living as a survivor.

Professional Issues and Service Implementation

Referral for Specialist Spiritual Assessment

A spiritual assessment is a formal evaluation of an individual's spiritual needs and resources conducted using the person's narrative, which includes meaning, purpose, and forgiveness. This specialized examination is carried out by trained spiritual care professionals.

In developed nations, most cancer programs have professional spiritual care providers or a care pathway for referral to trained chaplains; however, most of these services are utilized in palliative and end-of-life care. A referral pathway to pastoral care in survivorship clinics is not documented in the lit-erature. Also, not all cultural and spiritual traditions have such professional care providers. In some traditions, people function as priests or healers at places of worship.

Training in Spiritual Care

Studies have reported that, despite 58% of cancer survivors wishing to discuss spirituality and spiritual concerns with their oncologists, only 5–7% of the oncologists actually discuss these issues with their patients.[4] Care plans should include referral criteria for specialist services like pastoral care or chaplaincy. Culturally appropriate spiritual care services should become standard. An interprofessional curriculum on spiritual care has been developed and implemented by the George Washington University Institute for Spirituality and Health (ISPEC; see "Further Reading"). This multidisciplinary curriculum includes modules on different aspects of spiritual distress, assessment, compassion, and meaning. The ISPEC also assesses the spirituality of healthcare professionals themselves, a crucial issue because, when helping others in spiritual distress, healthcare professionals should be self-aware and comfortable with their own spirituality.

Vachon, in her narrative review on spirituality and meaning in cancer survivors, has elaborated on the implications for nurses about exploring spiritual issues with those cancer survivors with whom they interact significantly.[3] The nurse's role can include offering a supportive and confidential environment in which to initiate discussions about survivors' spiritual beliefs, concerns, and strategies, and the nurse can suggest referral to spiritual specialists.

Policies and Protocols

Most institutions in Western countries will have formal policies around referral to pastoral care and chaplaincy services. These programs are organized following a nondenominational spiritual model intended to be acceptable for cancer survivors of different ethnicities and religious backgrounds.

Conclusion

In summary, spirituality in cancer survivors affects their emotions, cognitions, social functioning, and quality of life, including their physical and mental health. Spiritual, religious, and existential issues are an integral part of the cancer survivor's journey as they move from illness to wellness; each step on this journey should focus on making meaning and purpose in life and on channeling their inner self and interpersonal relationships and connections to nature or a higher power. Oncology professionals should assess these myriad issues in a culturally sensitive manner and incorporate them into holistic survivorship care plans. Including spirituality in survivorship programs will go a long way toward ameliorating the long-term physical, emotional, social, and financial adversities that this vulnerable group faces in their lives.

Acknowledgments

I would like to express my deepest gratitude to Dr. Mark Lazenby for his guidance and mentorship.

References

1. Puchalski CM. Spirituality in the cancer trajectory. Ann Oncol. 2012;23(Suppl 3):iii49–iii55. doi: 10.1093/ANNONC/MDS088.

2. Winkelman WD, Lauderdale K, Balboni MJ, et al. The relationship of spiritual concerns to the quality of life of advanced cancer patients: Preliminary findings. 2011;14(9):1022–1028. doi: 10.1089/JPM.2010.0536. https://home.liebertpub.com/jpm.

3. Vachon MLS. Meaning, spirituality, and wellness in cancer survivors. Semin Oncol Nurs. 2008;24(3):218–225. doi: 10.1016/j.soncn.2008.05.010.

4. Nolan TS, Browning K, Vo JB, Meadows RJ, Paxton RJ. Assessing and managing spiritual distress in cancer survivorship. Am J Nurs. 2020;120(1):40. doi: 10.1097/01.NAJ.0000652032.51780.56.

5. Christian N, Broby T, Dorthe Olsen A, Børge J, Hvidt A. Spiritual, religious, and existential concerns of cancer survivors in a secular country with focus on age, gender and emotional challenges. doi: 10.1007/s00520-019-04775-4.

6. Cannon AJ, Darrington DL, Reed EC, Loberiza FR. Spirituality, patients' worry, and follow-up health-care utilization among cancer survivors. J Support Oncol. 2011;9(4):141–148. doi: 10.1016/J.SUPONC.2011.03.001.

7. Lewis PE, Sheng M, Rhodes MM, Jackson KE, Schover LR. Psychosocial concerns of young African American breast cancer survivors. J Psychosoc Oncol. 2012;30(2):168–184. doi: 10.1080/07347332.2011.651259.

8. Sabado M, Tanjasiri SP, alii SM, Hanneman M. Role of spirituality in coping with breast cancer: A qualitative study of Samoan breast cancer survivors and their supporters. Calif J Health Promot. 2010;8(SE):11. https://pmc.ncbi.nlm.nih.gov/articles/PMC3774055/

9. Munoz AR, Kaiser K, Yanez B, et al. Cancer experiences and health-related quality of life among racial and ethnic minority survivors of young adult cancer: A mixed methods study. Support Care Cancer. 2016;24(12):4861–4870. doi: 10.1007/S00520-016-3340-X.

10. U.S. Department of Health and Human Services, Office of Minority Health. National standards for culturally and linguistically appropriate services in health care: executive summary[Internet]. Rockville (MD): Office of Minority Health;2001 [cited 2025 Jan1], 13p. Available from: http://www.omhrc.gov/assest/pdf/checked/executive/pdf.

11. Deodar J, Park C, Lazenby M. Spiritually sensitive care in palliative and end of life settings: Psycho-oncology in palliative and end of life care. 2022. doi: 10.1093/MED/9780197615935.003.0009.

12. Riba MB, Donovan KA, Andersen B, et al. Distress management, version 3.2019: NCCN clinical practice guidelines in oncology. J Natl Comp Cancer Network. 2019;17(10):1229–1249. doi: 10.6004/JNCCN.2019.0048.

13. Puchalski CM. The FICA spiritual history tool #274. J Palliat Med. 2014;17(1):105–106. doi: 10.1089/JPM.2013.9458.

14. Anandarajah G, Hight E. Spirituality and medical practice: Using the HOPE questions as a practical tool for spiritual assessment. Am Fam Physician. 2001;63(1):81–88. doi: 10.1016/S1443-8461(01)80044-7.

15. Paloutzian RF, Agilkaya-Sahin Z, Bruce KC, et al. The Spiritual Well-Being Scale (SWBS): Cross-cultural assessment across 5 continents, 10 languages, and 300 studies. Assessing Spirituality in a Diverse World. December 7, 2020. doi: 10.1007/978-3-030-52140-0_17.

16. Peterman AH, Fitchett G, Brady MJ, Hernandez L, Cella D. Measuring spiritual well-being in people with cancer: The functional assessment of chronic illness therapy: Spiritual Well-being Scale (FACIT-Sp). Ann Behav Med. 2002;24(1):49–58. doi: 10.1207/S15324796ABM2401_06.

17. Daaleman TP, Frey BB. The Spirituality Index of Well-Being: A new instrument for health-related quality-of-life research. Ann Fam Med. 2004;2(5):499. doi: 10.1370/AFM.89.

18. Monod SM, Rochat E, Büla CJ, Jobin G, Martin E, Spencer B. The spiritual distress assessment tool: An instrument to assess spiritual distress in hospitalised elderly persons. BMC Geriatr. 2010;10:88. doi: 10.1186/1471-2318-10-88.

19. Gielen J, Kashyap K, Singh SP, Bhatnagar S, Chaturvedi SK. Psychometric assessment of SpiDiscl: Spiritual distress scale for palliative care patients in India. Indian J Palliat Care. 2022;28(1):13–20. doi: 10.25259/IJPC_50_21.

20. Yi JC, Syrjala KL. Anxiety and depression in cancer survivors. Med Clin North Am. 2017;101(6):1099. doi: 10.1016/J.MCNA.2017.06.005.

21. American Psychiatric Association. *Diagnostic and Statistical Manual of Mental Disorders.* American Psychiatric Association; 2013. doi: 10.1176/appi. books.9780890425596.x00diagnosticclassification.

22. Clarke DM, Kissane DW. Demoralization: Its phenomenology and importance. Austral N Z J Psychiatry. 2002. doi: 10.1046/j.1440-1614.2002.01086.x.

23. Wang Z, Xu D, Yu S, et al. Effectiveness of meaning-centered interventions on existential distress and mental health outcomes in cancer survivors and their family caregivers: A systematic review and meta-analysis of randomized controlled trials. Worldviews Evid Based Nurs. 2025;22(1). doi: 10.1111/WVN.12752.

24. Wei D, Liu XY, Chen YY, Zhou X, Hu HP. Effectiveness of physical, psychological, social, and spiritual intervention in breast cancer survivors: An integrative review. Asia Pac J Oncol Nurs. 2016;3(3):226–232. doi: 10.4103/2347-5625.189813.

25. Okere CA, Kvist T, Sak-Dankosky N, Yerris V. Spiritual interventions: Improving the lives of colorectal cancer survivors: A systematic literature review. J Adv Nurs. 2024;80(12). doi: 10.1111/JAN.16196.

26. Bernacchi V, LeBaron V, Porter K, Zoellner J, DeGuzman P. Barriers and facilitators to resilience for rural cancer survivors during COVID-19. Public Health Nurs. 2023;40(5):595–602. doi: 10.1111/PHN.13200.

27. Ownby KK. Use of the distress thermometer in clinical practice. J Adv Pract Oncol. 2019;10(2):175. https://pmc.ncbi.nlm.nih.gov/articles/PMC6750919/.

28. Thomas LPM, Meier EA, Irwin SA. Meaning-centered psychotherapy: A form of psychotherapy for patients with cancer. Curr Psychiatry Rep. 2014;16(10):488. doi: 10.1007/S11920-014-0488-2.

29. van der Spek N, Vos J, van Uden-Kraan CF, et al. Effectiveness and cost-effectiveness of meaning-centered group psychotherapy in cancer survivors: Protocol of a randomized controlled trial. BMC Psychiatry. 2014;14(1):1–8. doi: 10.1186/1471-244X-14-22/TABLES/2.

30. Mathew A, Doorenbos AZ, Jang MK, Hershberger PE. Acceptance and commitment therapy in adult cancer survivors: A systematic review and conceptual model. J Cancer Surviv. 2021;15(3):427–451. doi: 10.1007/S11764-020-00938-Z.

31. Jones RA, Taylor AG, Bourguignon C, et al. Complementary and alternative medicine modality use and beliefs among African American prostate

cancer survivors. Oncol Nurs Forum. 2007;34(2):359–364. doi: 10.1188/07.ONF.359-364.

32. Bastian TD, Burhansstipanov L. Sharing wisdom, sharing hope: Strategies used by Native American cancer survivors to restore quality of life. JCO Glob Oncol. 2020;6(6):161–166. doi: 10.1200/JGO.19.00215.

33. Singh-Carlson S, Wong F, Martin L, Nguyen SKA. Breast cancer survivorship and South Asian women: Understanding about the follow-up care plan and perspectives and preferences for information post treatment. Curr Oncol. 2013;20(2):e63-79. doi: 10.3747/CO.20.1066

Further Reading and Resources

Interprofessional Spiritual Care Education Curriculum (ISPEC™) | GWish | GW School of Medicine and Health Sciences. Accessed July 8, 2025. https://gwish.smhs.gwu.edu/programs/transforming-practice-health-settings/interprofessional-spiritual-care-education-curriculum-ispecc

Paloutzian RF, Park CL. *Handbook of the Psychology of Religion and Spirituality.* 2nd ed. Guilford Press; 2013.

Textbook examining psychological dimensions of spirituality.

Puchalski C, Jafari N, Buller H, Haythorn T, Jacobs C, Ferrell B. Interprofessional spiritual care education curriculum: A milestone toward the provision of spiritual care. J Palliat Med. 2020; 23(6):777–784. https://doi.org/10.1089/jpm.2019.0375

Recommended curriculum to train spiritual care providers.

Chapter 9

Childhood, Adolescent, and Young Adult Cancer Survivors

Lori Wiener, Claire E. Wakefield, Anne Maas, and Anne-Sophie Darlington

Learning Objectives

After reading this chapter, the clinician will be able to:

1. Understand and differentiate survivorship issues for childhood, adolescent, and young adult cancer survivors.
2. Identify developmentally relevant aspects of survivorship outcomes.
3. Explore interventions to improve psychosocial outcomes for young survivors.
4. Identify gaps to enhance quality of care in the future.
5. Understand relevant professional, ethical, and cultural issues for managing survivorship care for young people.

Background Evidence

Childhood, adolescent, and young adult cancer survivors face a significantly increased risk of developing late side effects of their cancers and cancer treatments (often termed "late effects"), with up to 60–90% experiencing chronic health conditions decades after treatment completion.[1] Late effects can include increased risk of developing second cancers, cardiovascular disease, endocrine and metabolic disorders, delayed sexual development and infertility, and dental problems, among many other challenges. The prevalence of chronic conditions increases over time, meaning that survivors require lifelong medical surveillance and intervention when late effects are identified. Alongside medical late effects, it is increasingly recognized through longitudinal studies and systematic reviews that survivors of childhood and adolescent cancers experience a poorer quality of life compared with similarly aged individuals without a cancer history. This includes emotional distress symptoms, mood and anxiety disorders, reduced achievement of expected educational and employment milestones and relationship outcomes, suicide risk, poor health behaviors, and increased overall mental health care service use.[2] Psychosocial challenges may be particularly pronounced during adolescence, a critical period for physical and psychological development marked by puberty, the formation of first relationships, and the discovery of one's sexuality. Fortunately, despite potential negative outcomes, young people also have a tremendous capacity for resilience and positive outcomes.[3]

Presenting Problems

Table 9.1 summarizes common presenting problems faced by families as young people transition into survivorship, their impacts and challenges, and considerations for the clinician.

Transition to Survivorship for the Whole Family

The whole family may rejoice at completing therapy, experiencing a renewed sense of hope for the future and pride in having reached this point in the cancer trajectory. At the same time, current frequent monitoring and fears associated with disease relapse and separation from the treatment team on whom the family has depended for so long may generate uneasiness in young patients and families. Additionally, there is often an expectation that families will transition to a life that resembled their life prior to the cancer diagnosis. Reorganizing family, work, school, and social lives takes time. The life that families envisioned prior to the cancer diagnosis may be quite different as well, in part due to changes in family priorities prior to cancer and because these young survivors may continue to experience physical symptoms and new deficits.

Significant fatigue is not unusual after treatment ends, hair may not have grown back, and many young survivors are likely to have physical scars and report a "foggy brain" along with trouble focusing. Some will be entering the nonmedical world with an amputated limb, and many will have experienced some medical trauma and the loss of (pre-cancer) friends and newer friends with cancer who did not survive. Adolescence and young adulthood are times for individuation, exploration of romantic relationships, and emotional growth, yet those who underwent cancer treatment during these formative years may find that they lack the social skills, independence, or coping skills necessary to re-engage with others their age. Despite these issues, preparing for the transition off treatment is often felt to be a missing component of overall cancer care.

✎ Key Point

Because survivors' risks of developing late side effects of their cancer treatment increase significantly over time, transition preparation and successful healthcare transition are critical to the long-term health of young survivors.

Transition to Adult Care

In most treatment centers, young survivors are required to transition from pediatric to adult healthcare as they enter adulthood. This transition can be challenging for young cancer survivors due to several interconnected factors,

Table 9.1 Summary of presenting problems from transition to survivorship

Presenting problem	Challenges faced by individuals and families	Considerations for the clinician
Transition to survivorship	All families experience considerable stress and disruption at this time, regardless of the prognosis This is often exacerbated by the loss of the care team that families relied upon during the patient's cancer treatment Families are required to quickly adapt to a new reality that can include: Loss of regular disease monitoring Hypervigilance of symptoms Anxiety around scans and investigations Difficulties reimagining a new "normal" Processing and adapting to the diagnosis and treatment experience Possible post-trauma symptoms for patients and/or parents	It is important to consider: • The stresses families have faced throughout the cancer trajectory • Prior coping, starting with learning about the diagnosis • Nonphysical impacts of cancer therapy such as distress, fatigue, cognitive impacts, and social isolation Families most at risk include: • Prior history of trauma and/or loss • Limited emotional or socioeconomic resources • Family and marital conflict, and families that have experienced separation • Parents who perceive themselves to be lone parenting
Transition to adult care	Transition to adult healthcare can be challenging for families of young survivors because: • The adult healthcare system may feel less supportive and personal than the pediatric healthcare system • Many families have developed deep attachments to their pediatric care team, making it difficult to transition to a new healthcare team • There may be a reduced focus on family-centered care in the adult setting, with an increased focus on the individual patient • Adult healthcare systems can appear more fragmented and less comprehensive than the care the family received in pediatrics • Patients and family must be made aware of the importance of increased advocating for their own health needs (compared to pediatric care)	Readiness for transition to adult care must consider each patient's unique developmental abilities and will be influenced by: • Location • Access to care • Health insurance coverage • Experiences of structural racism and subsequent health disparities Best practice transition preparation should include: • Provision of medical education • Assessment of life goals (e.g., education/career plans may need to be reconsidered) • Addressing any accumulated financial debt (a financial navigator or social worker may be able to assist) • Considerations of cultural, language, and spiritual factors, including training for culturally competent care to address sensitive issues (e.g., sexual health post-treatment) along with attention to unconscious biases that can influence healthcare providers' decisions and assessments

summarized in Table 9.1. A multifaceted response to transition is often required, one that allows for a seamless continuation from child/adolescent-centered to adult-oriented healthcare in a way that considers typical developmental processes at this stage of life as well as access, appropriateness, and continuity of healthcare services. A growing number of cancer centers have developed adolescent and young adult (AYA) programs. These interdisciplinary programs address the unique challenges AYAs face throughout their disease trajectory, including the transition from adolescent to adult care.

To improve organizational healthcare transition practices, the US Center for Health Care Transition (Got Transition; https://www.gottransition.org/) developed and disseminated six core elements of Health Care Transition (HCT) that offer a framework for clinicians and institutions to provide a structured transition process with patients and their caregivers, beginning early in adolescence and continuing into young adulthood. The six core elements are provided in Figure 9.1.

If cancer treatment is completed during childhood, development of basic transition skills should start approximately at age 12. For all survivors, transition skills include young people becoming increasingly comfortable meeting with healthcare clinicians without a caregiver present. Essential to a successful transition is the provision of health-related information that empowers and prepares young survivors to understand and communicate their own healthcare needs. As adolescents begin to exert more control over their lives and strive for independence from their family and treatment teams, they may become less adherent to recommended medical surveillance, especially after treatment ends. Preparing for transition includes an understanding of their cancer treatment, medications (purpose and dosages), costs associated with their care, and how to access medical and psychological support. Prearranged visits to adult units or survivorship clinics prior to leaving the pediatric setting can be especially useful.

The provision of a survivorship care plan that is tailored to the young person's clinical and personal needs is an important component of transition planning.[4] This includes explaining the meaning of the word "cure," what follow-up care (such as blood work, scans) will entail, and symptoms that should be reported immediately. Research suggests that survivorship care plans can improve clinic workflow, application of guidelines in clinical practice, and survivor shared decision-making.[5]

A major contribution to the field was the publication of the first set of 15 evidence-based pediatric psychosocial standards of care.[6] These provide a blueprint regarding what families need for optimal outcomes throughout the cancer trajectory. Those most critical for survivorship include:

- Psychosocial assessment (see Appendix B, "AYA Additional Screening Tools")
- Monitoring of neuropsychological outcomes
- Psychosocial follow-up in survivorship
- Assessment of financial burden and school re-entry

Although there is not yet an equivalent set of global standards for AYA cancer survivors, multiple clinical practice guidelines can support the delivery of best-practice psychosocial care for survivors of AYA cancer.[7]

SIX CORE ELEMENTS™ APPROACH AND TIMELINE FOR
YOUTH TRANSITIONING FROM PEDIATRIC TO ADULT HEALTH CARE

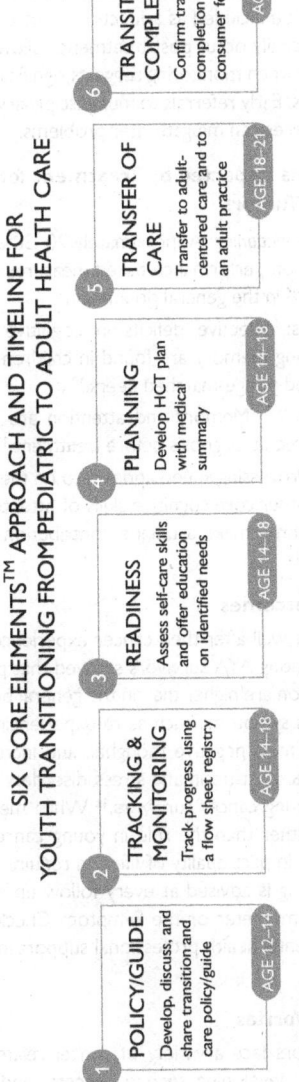

1 POLICY/GUIDE
Develop, discuss, and share transition and care policy/guide
AGE 12–14

2 TRACKING & MONITORING
Track progress using a flow sheet registry
AGE 14–18

3 READINESS
Assess self-care skills and offer education on identified needs
AGE 14–18

4 PLANNING
Develop HCT plan with medical summary
AGE 14–18

5 TRANSFER OF CARE
Transfer to adult-centered care and to an adult practice
AGE 18–21

6 TRANSITION COMPLETION
Confirm transfer completion and elicit consumer feedback
AGE 18–23

Figure 9.1 Six core elements for transitioning youth to adult health care.

Neurocognitive Considerations

Among the earliest and most widely recognized late effects of child and AYA cancer are neuropsychological deficits, particularly deficits in memory, metacognition, visuospatial/motor skills, and processing speed.[8] Difficulties in specific cognitive domains are associated with reduced quality of life, and potential deficits should be monitored during and after treatment. Academic achievement should be included as a functional outcome. A comprehensive assessment should ideally occur post-treatment, followed by a reassessment at 2–3 years later or when monitoring suggests significant neuropsychological or functional changes. Early referrals to multidisciplinary and interprofessional supportive care services can mitigate later problems.

Cognitive Domains Impacted by Treatment for Central Nervous System Tumors

- *Global intellectual functioning*: Approximately 20–30% of survivors demonstrate impairment on performance-based measures of intellect compared to the expected 2% in the general population.[9]
- *Executive functions*: Selective deficits in cognitive efficiency, problem-solving, and working memory are found in children treated for medulloblastoma compared to age-matched peers.[10]
- *Memory and attention*: Memory and attention are the principal domain found to be impaired at diagnosis before treatment.[11]
- *Processing speed*: Processing speed appears to be the central cognitive skill that disrupts the other core cognitive skills of attention span and working memory, and all three make a unique contribution to IQ and academic achievements.[8]

Mental Health Outcomes

Most survivors adapt well after their cancer experience.[12] However, a large systematic review among AYA survivors showed that psychological distress, anxiety, and depression are higher than in the general population.[13] Although post-traumatic stress symptoms such as re-experiencing trauma, avoidance of trauma-related stimuli, negative thoughts, and increased arousal have a prevalence of 2–20%, post-traumatic stress disorders (PTSD) remain relatively rare among young cancer survivors.[12] While mental health disorders are the exception rather than the rule in young cancer survivors, psychological challenges can impact quality of life and require intervention. Regular psychological screening is advised at every follow-up visit, using tools such as the Distress Thermometer or the Symptom Checklist-90, with referral pathways offering mental health professional support including cognitive behavioral therapy.[14]

Cancer-Related Worries

Young cancer survivors face a variety of cancer-related worries, including fears of recurrence, developing second cancers, and worries about late effects, infertility, and the health of their offspring. Fear of cancer recurrence is one of the most common challenges in this population. While awareness of cancer-related risks can encourage vigilance and adherence to health screenings, excessive worry can reduce quality of life and lead to maladaptive behaviors, such as excessive reassurance-seeking or avoidance of medical check-ups, both of which can have negative consequences. Inquiring about and addressing these worries is crucial (see also Chapter 3).

Families often find themselves surprised by periods of heightened anxiety after treatment ends. They appreciate being informed that these can be common, such as when the child presents with physical symptoms that remind them of the initial diagnosis (e.g., fevers, fatigue) or prior to monitoring scans. They also find it helpful to learn that anxiety usually decreases gradually after therapy as months pass and the young person remains disease-free. A range of psychological and physical interventions, such as cognitive behavioral therapy (CBT), relaxation techniques, and acceptance and commitment therapy (ACT) have shown promise in mitigating fear of recurrence, although most techniques have been studied in adult populations. The development and use of validated tools are crucial for assessing cancer-related worries. Promising measures include the Fear of Cancer Recurrence Inventory and the Cancer Worry Scale (see Appendix B).

Survivor Guilt

Cancer survivors may experience *survivor guilt*, which can lead them to feel ashamed of their own emotions, such as grief, sadness, or anger, especially when comparing their situation to others with cancer their age who have suffered more or did not survive. Consequently, some survivors may dismiss their own challenges, believing they have no right to complain and should instead be grateful for surviving. Oncology professionals should be aware of these emotional responses because they may lead young survivors to struggle with finding meaning in their continued existence.

While specific assessment tools and evidence-based interventions targeting survivor guilt in young cancer survivors are limited, normalizing these emotions and creating opportunities for emotional processing are widely endorsed in clinical practice. Interventions such as peer support groups, social support from loved ones, and professional counseling are frequently recommended and have shown general benefits in enhancing emotional well-being in cancer survivors.[15]

Post-Traumatic Growth

While young cancer survivors can face negative impacts from their illness, positive consequences, such as greater self-knowledge, a sense of having become a stronger person, the development of stronger interpersonal relationships, and a deeper appreciation for life have also been reported. These aspects are characteristics of post-traumatic growth (PTG). Research indicates that PTG in childhood cancer survivors is more common in those who are older at diagnosis, suggesting that a certain level of cognitive and emotional development is necessary to experience PTG.[12]

Positive and negative impacts of cancer do not fall on opposite ends of a continuum but can coexist in the same person at the same time. Healthcare practitioners should acknowledge both positive and negative consequences and that the presence of PTG does not imply the absence of mental health challenges in survivors.

Body Image

Research shows that AYA cancer survivors experience more body image issues compared to younger children with cancer and peers without a history of cancer.[16] Survivors have reported feeling unattractive, self-conscious, and worried when exposing scars, particularly during intimate situations.[17] For these individuals, supportive relationships appear instrumental in fostering body confidence.

Few assessment tools have been specifically developed for young cancer survivors. For survivors struggling with body image issues, interventions such as CBT, psycho-education, strength training, and physical exercise can be beneficial, although evidence specific to the young cancer survivor population is limited. As body image issues frequently co-occur with psychological distress and sexual dysfunction, it is important to offer integrated support that addresses these challenges.

Peer and Romantic Relationships

Peer relationships are crucial in supporting identity development and self-worth. Young cancer survivors report experiencing challenges in being able to maintain and form new friendships, feeling different from others, feeling embarrassed, and having trouble disclosing their previous diagnosis due to a fear of being misunderstood. Young survivors may feel isolated from peers during treatment and find that their experiences lead to either a sense of immaturity (missing developmental milestones) or a sense of increased maturity compared to peers, which can further hinder their ability to connect with others.

Romantic relationships play a crucial role in the lives of many adolescents and young adults who have survived cancer. Most young adult cancer survivors report satisfaction and positive outcomes from being in a relationship during and after treatment, finding comfort and support in their partners. Experience around forming intimate and romantic relationships, however, can be severely disrupted for preteens, adolescents, and young adults. This may lead young survivors to feel they lack certain skills and the confidence to engage in dating. Along with a fear of disease recurrence, many describe having a negative body image and worry about disclosing their cancer diagnosis, sexual dysfunction, and possible infertility to potential partners.[17]

Early and upfront communication is important in developing romantic relationships. Therefore, supporting and educating survivors in how and when to communicate experiences, worries, and insecurities can be beneficial. Needs assessments, such as the Childhood Cancer Survivor Study Needs Assessment Questionnaire (CCSS-NAQ), help to identify areas where survivors may benefit from targeted support, including relational and communication skills[18] (see Appendix B).

Sexual Health and Intimacy

Cancer survivors, particularly those diagnosed during adolescence and young adulthood, may face a variety of sexual health challenges, which vary based on their treatment and developmental stage. Adolescents and young adults in their early 20s often face interruptions in psychosexual development, leading to delays in sexual experiences compared to their peers. These interruptions can result in feelings of falling behind with social and sexual milestones, which may affect their confidence and relationships. Conversely, survivors in their late 20s or 30s, while typically less concerned with delayed psychosexual development, are more likely to encounter direct sexual dysfunction.[17] The impact of cancer and its treatment can lead to issues such as hormonal fluctuations, fatigue, perceived threats to femininity or masculinity, decreased libido, pain during intercourse, and anxiety about sexual performance. Research indicates that between 42% and 52% of survivors report at least one problem with sexual function, with overall sexual functioning being poorer compared to population norms.[17]

🔑 Key Point

Survivors consistently report a lack of sexual health discussions or guidance from healthcare providers and a desire for providers to address these issues. Open communication with partners and healthcare providers is crucial. Cancer survivors may benefit from medical and/or psychological assistance, including medical assessment and intervention (e.g., testosterone or estrogen supplementation, pelvic floor physical therapy), or psychosexual counseling to address their concerns.

Fertility

Young adulthood involves decisions about having children and planning for future family life. Cancer and its treatment can have lasting effects on reproductive health, and participation in fertility preservation varies based on available options. Fertility concerns can lead to feelings of loss and pressure to make decisions. Survivors also describe concerns about passing on a genetic risk of cancer to offspring. Uncertainty about fertility is associated with psychological distress, depression, and anxiety. Additionally, worries about fertility can adversely affect self-confidence and body image. Survivors may fear that infertility will impact their attractiveness as a partner and their future romantic relationships due to societal expectations regarding parenthood. Young cancer survivors with concerns about infertility often desire fertility status assessments and can benefit from referral to a reproductive specialist for further assessment. Psychological support is essential following a fertility status assessment.

If significant infertility risks are identified and survivors have a strong desire for parenthood, alternative family-building methods like adoption or surrogacy should be discussed. Psychologists can play a critical role in managing reproductive distress and exploring options as part of multidisciplinary survivorship care.

Interplay between Body Image, Relationships, and Sexual Function

Body image, romantic relationships, and sexual function are interconnected. A negative body image can affect a survivor's romantic relationships, while sexual dysfunction may stem from body image issues, which in turn can lead to difficulties within romantic relationships. Additionally, concerns about infertility can influence all three areas, highlighting the complex interplay between these aspects of a survivor's life.[17]

Financial Impact

There is growing awareness of the widespread and often devastating financial impact of cancer on families.[19] The true scale of the financial impact of cancer can become most apparent post-treatment, when families attempt to return to their previous lives. On top of facing the medical and nonmedical costs of cancer treatment (which can be high even in countries with universal healthcare programs), caregivers have often experienced major disruptions to their work, including reduced work hours; taken significant periods of leave; and missed opportunities for promotion, reskilling, and professional development. It can take many years for families to recover financially, with some choosing to deprioritize career development in the long term to spend more time on new priorities such as spending time together as a family.

Evidence shows that young survivors themselves are also at risk of long-term financial difficulties, including facing additional costs to secure health or life insurance, mortgages, and loans; experiencing more challenges in maintaining employment; and managing significant healthcare costs associated with ongoing cancer surveillance and management of late side effects of their cancer treatment. Multilevel interventions to alleviate financial toxicity in survivors of childhood and AYA cancer are urgently needed to tackle structural influences (e.g., government policy, insurance access, employer support) as well as individual influences (e.g., direct financial assistance, financial advice, vocational training) on survivors' and families' financial well-being. Timely support can include referral to vocational counseling to identify suitable employment options for young survivors' skills and abilities, as well as support from social workers and other professionals regarding benefits advice, employment guidance, and financial management.

Case Study

Sandra was diagnosed with Ewing's sarcoma at age 12 and treated with intensive chemotherapy, including drugs known to confer risk of long-term heart problems in some patients. She dropped out of university in her first year because she felt unable to relate to her peers and her "brain just feeling sluggish." She is now 23, living at home, and working as a manager of a coffee shop. This is a job she had enjoyed until a younger and newer employee received a promotion that she felt she deserved. Her two brothers have graduate degrees. She was referred for psychological assessment after a recent breakup and having shared what her mother described as suicidal thoughts. She is also being assessed for a cardiac condition.

Sandra easily engaged with the psychologist during their first few sessions. She spoke of being easily fatigued, angry about having a possible heart condition "after everything I have already been through," and feeling irritable and sad since her boyfriend of 9 months broke up with her. She described her cancer experience as "never ending" because people frequently ask her about the scars on her chest from multiple in-dwelling catheters; she was worried that she may never be able to have children, that her hair would never grow back as thick as it once was, and that now she had to go to "adult doctors that I don't like" for problems related to her childhood cancer treatment. Plus, she said, "It can even come back again!" She described being disappointed with herself since she does not earn enough money to move out of her parents' home and often feels her parents are disappointed in her. Sandra admitted that there are days when she is not sure "it is all worth it," but denied any self-harm behaviors, previous suicide attempts, or current thoughts of ending her life.

When asked about the hardest part of her cancer experience, Sandra teared up and shared recalling the day that she learned that a good friend from the hospital, who also had Ewing's sarcoma, died. She vividly recalled where she was in the hospital when learning this and then stated, "Wow, maybe this was even harder on me than I ever thought. That was a long time ago."

Points to Consider

- While Sandra exhibits symptoms of sadness and irritability, her symptom profile did not meet the criteria for a major depressive episode (differential diagnoses to consider are presented below). If she had not been referred for appropriate intervention, her mood difficulties may have worsened.

- Survivors may find themselves recalling and even re-experiencing some aspect of their childhood illness, which can complicate efforts to cope, particularly when faced with a new illness. Interventions such as CBT and ACT can be useful in mitigating this stress.

- Consider the emotional and physical sequelae from the cancer experience and ongoing medical concerns, especially as finding and maintaining employment can be a challenge for some young survivors. Employment is an important determinant of quality of life and has significant implications for independence, self-esteem, family and social relationships, and, in some settings, health insurance coverage

- Consider the dynamic relationship between medical, neurocognitive, and psychosocial issues that can impact quality of life (loss of a relationship, poor work performance, lack of independence).

- Address the disconnect between people's perceptions of what survivorship "should" look like and survivors' lived reality, along with the assumption that survivors should feel grateful.

- Explore the possible loss of former identity and life goals and whether there is a need to adjust to new or different possibilities for the future.

⚠ Immediate referral to a mental health specialist is indicated if survivors are identified as experiencing severe mental health difficulties (e.g., severe depression or psychosis), suicidal ideation or self-harming behaviors.

Investigations for Key Differential Diagnoses

- *Adjustment disorder:* The presence of emotional or behavioral symptoms in response to an identifiable stressor(s) such as hospital admissions that begin to occur within 3 months of the onset of the stressor(s).
- *Major depressive disorder:* A depressed mood that is present most of the day, nearly every day. This mood can be subjective, such as feeling hopeless or empty, or it can be observed by others.
- *Dysthymia:* Chronic persistent unhappiness for more days than not, as indicated by subjective account or observation by others, for at least 2 years.
- *Generalized anxiety disorder:* Excessive anxiety and worry about a number of activities or events (such as work and school performance), occurring more days than not for 6 months or longer.
- *Phobia:* Intense, irrational fear of specific situations, such as medical appointments or needles; these situations are then avoided or endured with intense fear or anxiety.
- *Post-traumatic stress disorder:* Trauma-related symptoms such as intrusive thoughts, flashbacks, and heightened arousal following a cancer diagnosis.
- *Somatic symptom disorder:* Excessive focus on and concern about physical symptoms such as pain, fatigue, weakness, or shortness of breath that are distressing or cause problems in daily life.
- *Obsessive-compulsive disorder:* Recurrent and persistent thoughts, urges, or images (such as the possibility of cancer recurrence) that are experienced as intrusive and unwanted.

Patient-Reported Outcome Measures

Early and ongoing psychosocial assessments are key to providing appropriate preventive interventions. Given the range of mental health challenges survivors may face, ongoing psychosocial monitoring is critical in survivorship care. Patient-reported outcome measures (PROMs) are increasingly used in clinical practice to assess survivors' psychosocial well-being through standardized, validated questionnaires (Table 9.2, and expanded in Appendix B). PROMs help to identify mental health issues, assess quality of life outcomes, and can improve communication between patients and doctors and improve patient satisfaction and self-management.[20] While discussing concerns with a clinician can help alleviate uncertainty for some survivors, those with significant psychosocial challenges typically benefit from referral to specialized care or interventions.

A recent international guideline harmonization project aimed to provide comprehensive guidance on surveillance of mental problems in survivors of child and AYA cancer noted that all healthcare providers should be aware that young survivors are at risk of developing mental health difficulties, including depression, anxiety, distress, post-traumatic stress, behavioral problems, and suicidal ideation.[2] Given this, some survivorship clinics are trialing routine administration of mental health screening tools (see Appendix A). However, each tool has limitations (e.g., limited language availability, problems assessed,

Table 9.2 Patient-reported outcome measures (PROMs) to assess major psychosocial issues

Psychosocial issue	Assessment tool[a]
Distress	Brief Symptom Inventory (BSI)-18
	Distress Thermometer (DT)
Post-traumatic stress	Posttraumatic stress response Diagnostic Scale (PDS)
Anxiety and depression	General Health Questionnaire (GHQ)
Cancer-related worries including fear of cancer recurrence	Cancer Worry Scale
	Fear of Cancer Recurrence Inventory (FCRI)
Quality of life	Generic/non–disease-specific: Pediatric Quality of Life Inventory (PedsQL)
	Cancer-related: Impact of Cancer-Childhood Survivors (IOC-CS)

[a]See Appendix B.

or costs), leading to the harmonization project providing example questions that could be tailored for use in different survivorship settings.

🔍 Key Point

Whichever screening tool is selected, routine psychosocial assessments should be followed by conversations with appropriate specialists or healthcare professionals to effectively address identified needs.

Pediatric Psychosocial Preventative Health Model

A major contribution to the field is the Pediatric Psychosocial Preventative Health Model (PPPHM), a three-tier biopsychosocial framework for assessing and treating families of children in the pediatric healthcare setting[21] (Figure 9.2).

The PPPHM matches level of need and risk to the type of interventions families might need. The largest group of families fall within the "universal" category. A smaller group of families fall within a "targeted" category—those at some elevated risk for ongoing psychosocial difficulties—while the smallest group of families in the "clinical" category exhibit more symptomatology and require the most treatment. The PPPHM model and the guidance that the psychosocial standards of care provide are useful throughout the cancer treatment trajectory and extending well into survivorship.

Clinical Management

Therapeutic Approaches

A range of psychotherapeutic approaches have been studied to support young survivors experiencing mental health difficulties, including CBT,

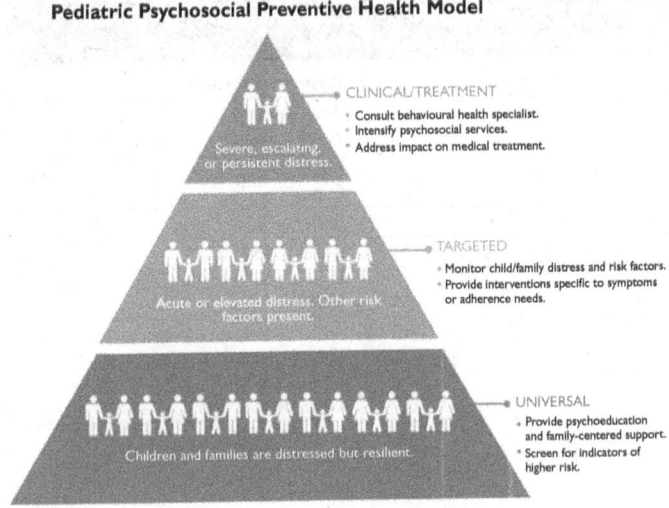

Figure 9.2 Pediatric psychosocial preventive health model.

mindfulness, family group therapy, social skills training, and music therapy, among other modalities.

- *Cognitive behavioral therapy* may be helpful in the treatment of anxiety, depression, and post-traumatic stress symptoms in childhood and AYA cancer survivors.
- *Family group therapy* has potential usefulness in ameliorating post-traumatic stress symptoms.
- *Music therapy* shows potential benefit in treating depression; however, there are few randomized trials assessing the efficacy of these approaches in young survivors, although more can be found in the adult literature.[2,12]
- *Telehealth*: Given that many young survivors face barriers to attending face-to-face psychosocial support programs (e.g., long travel times to treating centers, travel costs, desire to avoid the hospital environment), many survivorship programs have trialed digital (telehealth) modalities to provide support, either delivered synchronously (i.e., "live" or in real time) or asynchronously (e.g., via apps or platforms that provide helpful content without "live" interaction). Some digital interventions also include both modalities (e.g., live interaction with a mental health specialist and/or other young cancer survivors, plus provision of more static psycho-educational content). Digital interventions trialed to date have targeted a wide range of areas of difficulty for survivors, including mental health, self-management, quality of life, health behaviors (e.g., physical activity, nutrition, smoking cessation), and social skills, with mixed results.[22]

Key Point

Evidence-based standard of care: Survivors of child and adolescent cancers should receive yearly psychosocial screening throughout their lifespan for adverse educational and/or vocational progress; social and relationship difficulties; distress, anxiety, and depression; and risky health behaviors.[23]

Therapeutic Group Programs

Specifically developed for young cancer survivors (offering a mix of face-face and online modalities), these have been tested in multiple settings with some success, including the Surviving Cancer Competently Program (SCCIP) and Heros Plus in the United States, FAMOS in Denmark, the OK Onco Program in the Netherlands, and Recapture Life in Australia. Although preliminary studies show promise, further research using rigorous trial designs is required to establish their efficacy, cost-effectiveness, and sustainability. A recent review also noted that it may be harder to achieve positive outcomes from psychosocial interventions in survivors of AYA cancer than in survivors of childhood cancer.[22]

Key Point

It is important to recognize that childhood and AYA cancer can have a ripple effect throughout the young person's family and caring circle.

It is not uncommon for parents, siblings, and even grandparents to also encounter mental health and other psychosocial difficulties after the young patient successfully completes cancer treatment (see also Chapter 6). In some cases, caregivers experience more distress than survivors themselves as they process their experiences of caring for their child. Caregivers' psychosocial needs should therefore also be considered, including referral to specialist mental health providers when indicated. Several interventions for caregivers of childhood and AYA cancer survivors have been developed and evaluated, although many of these interventions are available only in particular settings or only through research trials. Similarly, there is a small selection of interventions (including camps) developed for siblings, but again these are often not easily accessible to all.[23]

Priority Populations

Subgroups of survivors are particularly vulnerable to psychosocial challenges including those diagnosed with central nervous system (CNS) tumors, those treated with cranial radiotherapy, and those reporting medical late effects (e.g., chronic graft versus host disease). Psychosocial challenges are also more common among female survivors and those with lower socioeconomic status. How survivors cope with their cancer experience, the meaning they assign to it, and the social support they receive play a crucial role in their psychological well-being. Moreover, parents often play a significant role in the lives of young survivors, and the psychological outcomes of parents and children are interconnected. Survivors whose parents experience distress are at a higher risk of psychological distress themselves and require intervention.[24]

Cultural Considerations

Across healthcare settings, young people and families from culturally and linguistically diverse (CALD) communities are also at increased risk of poor outcomes, including young people affected by cancer.[25] CALD families can face unique barriers to accessing high-quality survivorship care, including a lack of patient education resources in their own language, limited consideration of any unique cultural aspects of their experience from their healthcare providers, and incomplete understanding of their local health system, often resulting in greater unmet needs, psychosocial distress, and reduced engagement in care.[26] Young survivors from Indigenous communities are also considered a priority population given evidence that they are particularly at risk of experiencing unmet needs, thus underscoring the importance of engaging with Indigenous communities and Indigenous medical liaison/navigator services wherever available.

Sexual and Gender Minorities

The sexual and gender minority population with cancer can experience poorer quality of life because of increased psychological distress, stigma, discrimination, feelings of exclusion, minority stress, more chronic conditions, and poorer cancer outcomes.

Low- and Middle-Income Countries

It is important to note that the majority of young cancer survivors live in low- and middle-income countries (LMICs), about whom there has been little research to date.[27] Evidence shows that young survivors in LMICs often face a significant burden of medical late effects, with major barriers to receiving best-practice survivorship care.

🔍 Key Point

These findings speak to the need for a team approach that is attentive to potential barriers to care, inclusivity, and the importance of patient navigation to facilitate care coordination.

Professional Issues and Service Implementation

Recording and Communication

Communication of sensitive information in an age-appropriate way and determining the amount of information to share presents problems for health professionals. Despite evidence-based psychosocial standards of care for young people with cancer, most medical professionals lack formal training in identifying and understanding psychosocial issues and, therefore, can miss opportunities to identify, record, and respond to psychosocial issues experienced by patients. Systematically scheduled assessments using tools with strong psychometrics are recommended (see Appendix B).

Coordination of Survivorship Care

Survivorship care can include oncologist-led follow-up, multidisciplinary survivorship clinics, shared care, and care led by primary care. This care can be restricted by lack of training for primary care providers, poor communication between services, and limited capacity within tertiary treatment centers. The close relationships healthcare providers form with patients and family members increases the likelihood of identifying and managing issues. While limited access to mental health professionals can impede management, connecting with community resources can be very helpful. Additional resources in the form of screening and assessment tools for child and AYA survivors can be found in Appendix B at the end of this book.

Common Ethical Dilemmas

Survivorship presents unique ethical challenges.[28] Ethical dilemmas generally center around infringing on autonomy, informed consent, the child's and young person's rights, and decisions around treatment. Within survivorship, ethical issues to be mindful of are related to autonomy, care refusal or abandonment, truth-telling, and fertility preservation. Conflicting perspectives that may impact decision-making also occasionally arise (e.g., child and parent disagreeing about treatment).

Teams and Supervision

Health professionals caring for young people and their families over the relatively long treatment trajectory may witness emotional and physical suffering, difficulties in managing symptoms, and, in some instances, the inability to cure patients. Providing psychosocial care to patients and families can be powerful, meaningful, and intimate as well as emotionally draining. These factors can lead to burnout, compassion fatigue, moral distress, and grief. A sense of loss can also occur after treatment is completed and patients and families transition to survivorship care. An ongoing multidisciplinary approach is essential to address both the medical and psychosocial effects of cancer diagnosed in younger patients and their families. Individual supervision can be critically important to address challenging cases as well as career development. When appropriate, confidential referral to counseling services can be made. Regularly scheduled team meetings can be useful for team building, case discussions, and professional trainings. Psychosocial rounds provide an opportunity for all staff members to plan together a coordinated approach to patient care. Well-being programs that include debriefing (e.g., debriefs with colleagues after critical events: "hot" debriefs occur immediately after the event, while "cold" debriefs occur after the event, to allow time for reflection and learning), wellness resources, and improved support and communication within teams can be helpful around staff retention and avoiding burnout.

References

1. *Late Effects of Treatment for Childhood Cancer (PDQ(R)): Health Professional Version*. PDQ Cancer Information Summaries; 2002.

2. Marchak JG, Christen S, Mulder RL, et al. Recommendations for the surveillance of mental health problems in childhood, adolescent, and young adult cancer survivors: A report from the International Late Effects of Childhood Cancer Guideline Harmonization Group. Lancet Oncol. 2022;23(4):e184–e196. doi: 10.1016/S1470-2045(21)00750-6.

3. Salsman JM, Rosenberg AR. Fostering resilience in adolescence and young adulthood: Considerations for evidence-based, patient-centered oncology care. Cancer. 2024;130(7):1031–140. doi: 10.1002/cncr.35182 [published Online First: 20240101].

4. Hill RE, Wakefield CE, Cohn RJ, et al. Survivorship care plans in cancer: A meta-analysis and systematic review of care plan outcomes. Oncologist. 2020;25(2):e351–e372. doi: 10.1634/theoncologist.2019-0184 [published Online First: 20191025].

5. King JE, O'Connor MC, Shohet E, et al. Clinician perceptions of Passport for Care, a web-based clinical decision support tool for survivorship care plan delivery. Pediatr Blood Cancer. 2023;70(1):e30070. doi: 10.1002/pbc.30070 [published Online First: 20221103].

6. Wiener L, Kazak AE, Noll RB, Patenaude AF, Kupst MJ. Standards for the psychosocial care of children with cancer and their families: An introduction to the special issue. Pediatr Blood Cancer. 2015;62(Suppl 5):S419–424. doi: 10.1002/pbc.25675 [published Online First: 20150923].

7. Bhatia S, Pappo AS, Acquazzino M, et al. Adolescent and Young Adult (AYA) Oncology, Version 2.2024, NCCN clinical practice guidelines in oncology. J Natl Compr Canc Netw. 2023;21(8):851–880. doi: 10.6004/jnccn.2023.0040.

8. Walsh KS, Noll RB, Annett RD, Patel SK, Patenaude AF, Embry L. Standard of care for neuropsychological monitoring in pediatric neuro-oncology: Lessons from the Children's Oncology Group (COG). Pediatr Blood Cancer. 2016;63(2):191–195. doi: 10.1002/pbc.25759 [published Online First: 20151009].

9. Brinkman TM, Krasin MJ, Liu W, et al. Long-term neurocognitive functioning and social attainment in adult survivors of pediatric CNS tumors: Results from the St Jude Lifetime Cohort Study. J Clin Oncol. 2016;34(12):1358–1367. doi: 10.1200/JCO.2015.62.2589 [published Online First: 20160201].

10. Law N, Smith ML, Greenberg M, et al. Executive function in paediatric medulloblastoma: The role of cerebrocerebellar connections. J Neuropsychol. 2017;11(2):174–200. doi: 10.1111/jnp.12082 [published Online First: 20150804].

11. Margelisch K, Studer M, Ritter BC, Steinlin M, Leibundgut K, Heinks T. Cognitive dysfunction in children with brain tumors at diagnosis. Pediatr Blood Cancer. 2015;62(10):1805–1812. doi: 10.1002/pbc.25596 [published Online First: 20150605].

12. Michel G, Brinkman TM, Wakefield CE, Grootenhuis M. Psychological outcomes, health-related quality of life, and neurocognitive functioning in survivors of childhood cancer and their parents. Pediatr Clin North Am. 2020;67(6):1103–1134. doi: 10.1016/j.pcl.2020.07.005 [published Online First: 20200923].

13. Osmani V, Horner L, Klug SJ, Tanaka LF. Prevalence and risk of psychological distress, anxiety and depression in adolescent and young adult (AYA) cancer survivors: A systematic review and meta-analysis. Cancer Med. 2023;12(17):18354–18367. doi: 10.1002/cam4.6435 [published Online First: 20230810].

14. Holmer P, Michel G, Dyntar D, Bolliger C. Screening for mental health problems in childhood cancer survivorship: A systematic review. Pediatr Blood Cancer. 2022;69:S401–S02.

15. Maas A, Maurice-Stam H, van der Aa-van Delden AM, et al. Positive and negative survivor-specific psychosocial consequences of childhood cancer: The DCCSS-LATER 2 psycho-oncology study. J Cancer Surviv. 2024;18(5):1505–1516. doi: 10.1007/s11764-023-01394-1 [published Online First: 20230511].

16. Vani MF, Lucibello KM, Trinh L, Santa Mina D, Sabiston CM. Body image among adolescents and young adults diagnosed with cancer: A scoping review. Psycho-Oncology. 2021;30(8):1278–1293. doi: 10.1002/pon.5698 [published Online First: 20210421].

17. Cherven BO, Demedis J, Frederick NN. Sexual health in adolescents and young adults with cancer. J Clin Oncol. 2024;42(6):717–724. doi: 10.1200/JCO.23.01390 [published Online First: 20231019].

18. Cox CL, Sherrill-Mittleman DA, Riley BB, et al. Development of a comprehensive health-related needs assessment for adult survivors of childhood cancer. J Cancer Surviv. 2013;7(1):1–19. doi: 10.1007/s11764-012-0249-3 [published Online First: 20121205].

19. Ruiz S, Hudson MM, Ehrhardt MJ, Maki J, Ackermann N, Waters EA. Childhood cancer survivors, financial toxicity, and the need for multilevel interventions. Pediatrics. 2023;152(1):e2022059951. doi: 10.1542/peds.2022-059951.

20. Leahy AB, Steineck A. Patient-reported outcomes in pediatric oncology: The patient voice as a gold standard. JAMA Pediatr. 2020;174(11):e202868. doi: 10.1001/jamapediatrics.2020.2868 [published Online First: 20201102].

21. Kazak AE, Schneider S, Didonato S, Pai AL. Family psychosocial risk screening guided by the Pediatric Psychosocial Preventative Health Model (PPPHM) using the Psychosocial Assessment Tool (PAT). Acta Oncol. 2015;54(5):574–580. doi: 10.3109/0284186X.2014.995774 [published Online First: 20150309].

22. Zhang A, Wang K, Zebrack B, Tan CY, Walling E, Chugh R. Psychosocial, behavioral, and supportive interventions for pediatric, adolescent, and young adult cancer survivors: A systematic review and meta-analysis. Crit Rev Oncol Hematol. 2021;160:103291.

23. Mooney-Doyle K, Burley S, Ludemann E, Rawlett K. Multifaceted support interventions for siblings of children with cancer: A systematic review. Cancer Nurs. 2021;44(6):E609–E635. doi: 10.1097/NCC.0000000000000966.

24. Sultan S, Leclair T, Rondeau E, Burns W, Abate C. A systematic review on factors and consequences of parental distress as related to childhood cancer. Eur J Cancer Care (Engl). 2016;25(4):616–637. doi: 10.1111/ecc.12361 [published Online First: 20150910].

25. Kasherman L, Yoon WH, Tan SYC, Malalasekera A, Shaw J, Vardy J. Cancer survivorship programs for patients from culturally and linguistically diverse (CALD) backgrounds: A scoping review. J Cancer Surviv. 2023. doi: 10.1007/s11764-023-01442-w [published Online First: 20230812].

26. Kim S, Cho J, Shin DW, Jeong SM, Kang D. Racial differences in long-term social, physical, and psychological health among adolescent and young adult cancer survivors. BMC Med. 2023;21(1):289. doi: 10.1186/s12916-023-03005-3 [published Online First: 20230804].

27. Wong KA, Moskalewicz A, Nathan PC, Gupta S, Denburg A. Physical late effects of treatment among survivors of childhood cancer in low- and middle-income

countries: a systematic review. J Cancer Surviv. 2025 Jun;19(3):1-17. doi: 10.1007/s11764-023-01517-8. Epub 2024 Jan 6. PMID: 38183576.

28. Sisk BA, Canavera K, Sharma A, Baker JN, Johnson LM. Ethical issues in the care of adolescent and young adult oncology patients. Pediatr Blood Cancer. 2019;66(5):e27608. doi: 10.1002/pbc.27608 [published Online First: 20190108].

Further Reading and Resources

Benedict C, Ahmad Z, Lehmann V, Ford JS. Sexual health, fertility, and relationships in cancer care. In: Watson M, Kissen D, eds. *Adolescents and Young Adults. Psycho-oncology Care Series: Companion Guides for Clinicians. Sexual Health, Fertility, and Relationships in Cancer Care.* Oxford University Press; 2020.

Bolliger C, Way K, Michel G, Sodergren SC, Darlington AS, EORTC Quality of Life Group. Mapping and comparing the quality of life outcomes in childhood and adolescent and young adult cancer survivors: An umbrella review and future directions. Quality of Life Research. 2024 Mar;34(3):633-656. doi: 10.1007/s11136-024-03825-7. Epub 2024 Dec 19. PMID: 39699829; PMCID: PMC11919941.

Bradford N, Chan RJ, Skrabal Ross X, et al. Childhood cancer models of survivorship care: a: A scoping review of elements of care and reported outcomes. J Cancer Surviv. 2024. doi: 10.1007/s11764-024-01610-6 [published Online First: 20240509].

COSA. COSA guidelines for the psychosocial management of AYAs diagnosed with cancer. 2024. https://www.cosa.org.au/media/5zaj2keg/cosa-aya-psychosocial-guidelines-public-consultation-draft-30-09-24.pdf

Devine KA, Christen S, Mulder RL, et al. Recommendations for the surveillance of education and employment outcomes in survivors of childhood, adolescent, and young adult cancer: A report from the International Late Effects of Childhood Cancer Guideline Harmonization Group. Cancer. 2022;128(13):2405–2419. doi: 10.1002/cncr.34215 [published Online First: 20220418].

Devine KA, Viola AS, Coups EJ, et al. Digital health interventions for adolescent and young adult cancer survivors. JCO Clin Cancer Inform. 2018;2:1–15.

White P, Schmidt A, Shorr J, Ilango S, Beck D, McManus M. *Six Core Elements of Health Care Transition™ 3.0.* Got Transition, The National Alliance to Advance Adolescent Health; July 2020.

Whitford B, Nadel AL, Fish JD. Burnout in pediatric hematology/oncology: Time to address the elephant by name. Pediatr Blood Cancer. 2018;65(10):e27244. doi: 10.1002/pbc.27244 [published Online First: 20180524].

WHO. Cancer in Children. Sept 2018. Available from: https://www.who.int/news-room/fact-sheets/detail/cancer-in-children. Accessed October 21, 2024.

Chapter 10

Psychosocial Considerations for Rehabilitation in Cancer Survivorship

Christoffer Johansen, Bogda Koczwara, and Wendy Lam

Learning Objectives

After reading this chapter, the clinician will be able to:

1. Recognize impacts and consequences of cancer treatments and common impairments that cancer survivors may experience.
2. Understand the role of psychosocial care in rehabilitation and prehabilitation in the context of cancer survivorship.
3. Consider the critical components of rehabilitation care and their implementation in diverse resource settings.
4. Understand the importance of early rehabilitation interventions, preferably beginning at the date of diagnosis.
5. Understand prehabilitation and its link to post-treatment rehabilitation.
6. Be aware of the need for a personal approach when offering rehabilitation to patients with cancer, such as socioeconomic factors, multimorbidity, prescribed drugs, lifestyle, and cultural background.

Background Evidence

The World Health Organization (WHO) defines rehabilitation as "interventions designed to optimize function and reduce disability in individuals with health conditions in their interaction with their environment" and sees it as an essential component of universal health coverage.[1] Within this definition, there is an explicit recognition of rehabilitation interventions[2,3] for individuals with cancer that address a range of needs,[4] including mental and cognitive function, pain, and physical and sexual function, as well as interpersonal relationships, educational and vocational needs, community life, lifestyle and exercise, self-management, and caregiver support.[5] Issues concerning return to work, anxiety and depression, and the needs of caregivers (often spouses or close family members) also are of importance.[6] The Package of Interventions for Rehabilitation (PIR) was developed by the WHO to address the global need for rehabilitation across 20 conditions with high prevalence and high levels of associated disability, including cancer. Many aspects of the WHO PIR align with the mission and focus of the International Psycho-Oncology Society (IPOS). The WHO PIR malignant neoplasm module highlights a range of areas for rehabilitation in people affected by cancer, spanning many of the above-mentioned functioning domains (see "Further Reading and Resources" section). These interventions, while commonly delivered during or after cancer treatment, may be initiated before cancer treatment commences to prevent impairment.[7]

Presenting Problems

No individual experiences cancer treatment without concurrently experiencing challenges arising from physiological malfunction in various parts of the body. In addition, psychological and social challenges occur, often in the form of inability to participate in activities that prior to the cancer diagnosis were a part of everyday life; such activities may be difficult to continue during and following treatment. Regardless of the target of the treatment, patients with cancer may experience a range of issues that require rehabilitation intervention. In a nationwide and population-based cohort study from Denmark, it was shown that every second patient with cancer was diagnosed with a chronic disease at the time of cancer diagnosis and that 35% fulfilled the criteria for polypharmacy, taking five or more different drugs every day.[8] Across cancer sites, most patients experience some level of fatigue during their course of treatment; however, approximately 30% of patients will be chronically fatigued for a number of years after treatment.[4] Based on a meta-analysis and review of studies on depression and anxiety, we know that approximately 20% of cancer survivors experience clinical depression within the first 5 years after diagnosis, and approximately 15% experience one clinical episode of anxiety requiring clinical intervention.[9] In addition, for some cancer patients return to work is of importance for several reasons including income, social networking, and quality of life. The issue of work and job satisfaction are influenced by national regulations and the organization of the jobs market but also by the introduction of new treatments that require more visits to hospitals. The topic of return to work is thoroughly presented in Chapter 7. Functional impairments in the form of late effects (e.g., a colostomy, lymphedema, or major depression) require specific interventions aiming at restoring function, and rehabilitation programs also provide surveillance for the vital early recognition of second cancers.[10] The need for rehabilitation programs to optimize functioning is incontrovertible.

General problems such as fatigue, pain, or depression are prevalent no matter which type of cancer treatment addresses. And, aside from such general problems, more specific problems arise from the organ or organ systems that the treatment targets; for example, if treatment is focused on a gynecological cancer, urination, defecation, diarrhea/constipation, and sexuality may require rehabilitation.

Among 4,512 cancer survivors in a study by the American Cancer Society, common symptoms included pain (e.g., backache, muscle ache), treatment-related symptoms (e.g., dry mouth, hair loss, paresthesia), fatigue, nausea and vomiting, bowel/bladder control problems, weight change, and lung symptoms (e.g., cough, dyspnea).[4] Other prevalent symptoms included poor sleep, mood change, and change in mental wellness.

The overall and site-specific incidence and time of prevalence of problems calling for rehabilitation is difficult to estimate because 50% of patients have pre-existing chronic illnesses. These general issues are accompanied by numerous more specific complaints, symptoms, and diseases that may affect the cancer survivor from the date of diagnosis and into the first years of survivorship (e.g., urinary leakage, lymphedema of arms or legs, cognitive dysfunction, sensory deficiencies, constipation/diarrhea, and reduction in cardiac functioning). Other pertinent problems include aspects of autonomy (e.g., independence, ability to obtain meaningfulness, ability to work and participate in recreational activities).

Investigations for Key Differential Diagnoses

Using the WHO PIR screening approach, assessment begins with a detailed interview listing comorbidities and the treatments provided for them as well as an entire medical history of possible exposures. Based on this interview, the clinician follows the flowchart listing key approaches to address the patient's problems (see Further reading and Resources section), these are then prioritized by information during this initial dialogue with the patient, in combination with an evaluation of known eventual comorbidities and the concurrent treatment of these comorbidities. Rehabilitation may include several initiatives to support the patient in gaining better overall health (e.g., light cardio training in combination with smoking cessation and reduction in alcohol intake or dietary planning). Such programs become more well-defined as the patient and clinician discuss and refine suggested lifestyle changes or lifestyle-based optimizations and interventions. Family members or close friends often play a major role in successful outcomes from lifestyle changes, and these individuals should be included in the assessment and planning phases. Additionally, it is important to recognize any potential interactions with the treatments administered by a hematologist or an oncologist.

Rehabilitation interventions typically take place in a hospital, but, following discharge to the local community, liaisons must be established between community services and highly specialized hospital departments. Such organizational and structural issues will depend on the local health system and the availability of community-based services that can provide rehabilitation. In areas without on-site rehabilitation facilities, it may be possible to organize telehealth personalized monitoring to help the patient maintain the required exercises or lifestyle changes suggested by their cancer care team. The WHO PIR interview provides a useful guide for determining the rehabilitation needs in the individual patient.

Needs Assessment Questionnaires

Rehabilitation or follow-up of cancer patients is ideally conducted by doctors, nurses, and other allied health disciplines (e.g., physiotherapists, dieticians, social workers) working in collaboration. An example of nurse-conducted clinical follow-up was demonstrated in one randomized trial among women with stage I and II breast cancer, showing that a follow-up conducted by nurses was superior to follow-up conducted by oncology specialists when patients had been trained in Guided Self-Determination (GSD).[11] GSD is an evidence-based method and a dialogue tool for mutual decision-making. Patient-centered in construction, it ensures that the patient and healthcare professionals cooperate from the outset on addressing whatever issues the patient experiences as most relevant and challenging. GSD in the health system involves reflection, cooperation, and change, helping patients and healthcare professionals to clarify and collaborate constructively about difficult health challenges. The follow-up in the above trial lasted 36 months, and the intervention group showed a significantly higher level of quality of life and significantly lower levels of depression, anxiety, and fear of recurrence. The women in the intervention group were provided with an opportunity to report and discuss symptoms, and the management of these symptoms, with project-assigned nurses at the hospital, illustrating one way of dealing with the daily challenges and rehabilitation needs of patients during cancer survivorship.[12] GSD encourages patients (and to some degree spouses) in initiating rehabilitation activities by introducing a way to cope with immediate problems in life following a cancer treatment.[13] The engagement of patients in rehabilitation choices and in specific initiatives and programs likely secures higher compliance with the content of rehabilitation programs compared to programs simply prescribed by the physician or another health professional.

Survivorship Care Plans (SCP) may be realized by creating a document listing several important actions to be carried out by the patient to ensure the highest quality of life in the survivorship period. The SCP connects the highly specialized hospital department with community health professionals (e.g., general practitioners, home or community nurses, and health centers located in municipalities). The SCP documents the disease, the treatment provided at the hospital, and the overall recommendations.

The Cancer Needs Assessment Tool (NAT-C)[14] is a structured form comprising five sections:
- Priority referral for further assessment (highlighting any need for palliative care referral)
- Patient well-being
- Ability of caregiver or family to care for the patient
- Caregiver/family well-being
- Resulting referrals (if required)

Where problems are identified, the tool encourages clinicians to report what action is taken. The NAT-C was developed in Australia and has been shown to reduce the unmet informational needs of cancer patients in the oncology clinic. This is one of several tools to secure both a broad holistic view of the patient and their specific situation in several domains of life.

Case Study

Mr. R. is a 58-year-old man with type 2 diabetes and stage III colorectal cancer who underwent a hemicolectomy with a temporary stoma (scheduled for reversal in 6–12 months) and 6 months of adjuvant chemotherapy. Following treatment completion, he developed peripheral neuropathy, likely attributable to both diabetes and chemotherapy, and he has experienced considerable distress regarding his stoma. This has resulted in social withdrawal and challenges in resuming his occupation as a shopkeeper.

Challenges:

Physical: Mr. R faces impaired mobility due to neuropathy, difficulties in stoma care, and fatigue.

Psychosocial: He experiences anxiety related to stoma care, depression stemming from social isolation, and concerns about body image that impact his self-esteem.

Vocational: He encounters difficulties with prolonged standing, managing the stoma at work, and uncertainty regarding the timeline for recovery.

Rehabilitation plan:

Physical: The plan includes physiotherapy to address neuropathy through balance exercises and strength training, as well as training in stoma care.

Psychosocial: Counseling is recommended to address adjustment issues, along with peer support for patients managing stomas and stress management techniques.

Vocational: Workplace adaptations are suggested, including temporary seated duties and flexible scheduling.

Outcome: The anticipated outcomes include improved mobility, increased confidence in stoma care, and full vocational reintegration.

Clinical Management

Global Perspectives

The WHO developed the PIR in 2023. The PIR presents evidence-supported rehabilitation interventions applicable to all impacted individuals across various service delivery levels. It places particular importance on its relevance to communities or countries with low- to middle-level resources. The PIR for cancer covers 14 functioning domains and 3 secondary condition domains, with a total of 26 related assessments and 48 interventions.[1] Many of the functioning domains in the PIR for cancer include psychosocial components for assessment and intervention (see Table 10.1).

Recently, the IPOS, which champions psychosocial cancer care as a fundamental right, published a commentary endorsing the WHO PIR for cancer.[15]

Table 10.1 Summary of content of World Health Organization package of intervention for malignant neoplasm (cancer) module highlighting the psychosocial aspects of rehabilitation

Area	Assessment	Interventions
Mental/cognitive functions	Fatigue	Physical exercise training
		Psychological therapies
	Sleep functions	Cognitive behavioral therapy
	Body image	Psychosocial interventions
	Cognitive functions	Cognitive training
		Physical exercise training
Pain management	Pain	Pharmacological treatments
		Transcutaneous electrical stimulation
		Thermotherapy
		Soft-tissue techniques
		Physical exercise training
		Relaxation training
		Cognitive behavioral therapy
Sexual functions and intimate relationships	Sexual function and intimate relationships	Pelvic floor exercises
Cardiovascular and immunological functions	Edema (including lymphedema)	Range of motion exercises
		Muscle-strengthening exercises
		Skin care
		Retrograde massage
		Provision and training in use of products for compression therapy
	Vasomotor symptoms (hot flashes, night sweating)	Antidepressants
		Cognitive behavioral therapy
Motor functions and mobility	Joint mobility	Range-of-motion exercises
	Muscle functions	Muscle-strengthening exercises
	Balance	Balance training
	Gait pattern and walking	Provision and training in use of assistive products for mobility
	Mobility (incl. fall risk)	Mobility training
		Provision and training in the use of assistive products for mobility
Exercise and fitness	Exercise capacity	Fitness training
Activities of daily living	Activities of daily living	Activities of daily living training
		Provision and training in use of assistive products for self-care
		Modification of the home environment

Table 10.1 Continued		
Area	**Assessment**	**Interventions**
Interpersonal interactions and relationships	Interpersonal interactions and relationships	Psychosocial interventions
Education and vocation	Educational assessment	Educational counseling, training, and support
	Vocational assessment	Vocational counseling, training, and support
Community and social life	Participation in community and social life	Participation focused interventions
Lifestyle modification	Lifestyle risk factors	Education, advice, and support for healthy lifestyle
Self-management	Self-efficacy, health and digital literacy, self-management supports	Education, advice, support for self-management
		Education and advice on self-directed exercise
Carer and family support	Carer and family needs	Carer and family training and support
Mental health (depression, anxiety, emotional distress)	Mental health	Antidepressants
		Psychological therapies (including cognitive behavioral therapy)
		Physical exercise training
		Stress management training

Adapted from the original WHO module. Sources: Package of interventions for rehabilitation. Module 1. Introduction. License: CC BY-NC-SA 3.0 IGO; and Package of interventions for rehabilitation. Module 7. Malignant neoplasm. World Health Organization; 2023. License: CC BY-NC-SA 3.0 IGO.

To effectively incorporate cancer-related psychosocial rehabilitation services into standard cancer treatment, it is essential to develop a model that can be sustained over time.

Despite growing evidence for the therapeutic effects of many psychosocial interventions highlighted in the PIR for cancer, its utility and sustainability in real-world settings have yet to be addressed. Therapist-led face-to-face psychosocial interventions are resource-intensive, limiting reach due to constrained health budgets and therapist shortages. An evidence-based cancer rehabilitative psychosocial care model is urgently needed to optimize intervention effectiveness with minimal resources. The stepped care model, which adjusts intervention intensity based on concern severity, offers a more accessible and cost-effective solution. High-intensity interventions should be reserved for those with significant unmet needs, while less intensive, digital, self-guided interventions should be initially offered to those with mild to moderate concerns, with an option to escalate for nonrespondents.

Prehabilitation

When is the right time for a cancer patient to begin working on lifestyle changes that may contribute to a better outcome for the interventions provided by surgeons, medical oncologists, radiation specialists, and allied health clinicians (e.g., physiotherapists, dieticians)? In recent years, research has emerged challenging the classic model of initiating rehabilitation following primary treatment, which thereby misses opportunities to achieve benefits for the patient by starting the rehabilitation at time of diagnosis. This more preventive approach has rehabilitation specialists meet patients at the time of diagnosis to begin interventions from which the patient may immediately benefit. Imagine a smoker having a tobacco-associated cancer diagnosed. What would be more relevant than to stop this smoking habit or, if not possible, reduce the daily smoking pattern? It has been shown in large cohorts of cancer patients that continuous smoking leads to early death compared to patients who cease smoking immediately.[16]

In most cases, before systemic treatment is initiated, some kind of surgery will take place, and it is in this field of prehabilitation research that we have the largest knowledge base.[17,18] Decreased alcohol consumption, healthy dietary changes, increased physical activity, and changes in or cessation of smoking habits entails a better outcome for cancer surgery.[17,19] Multimodal prehabilitation interventions before cancer surgery may reduce hospital stay and lower complication rates particularly in older cancer patients. And, in considering all abdominal and thoracic cancers undergoing surgery, both preoperative and perioperative physiotherapy is likely to reduce the incidence of postoperative lung complications. Further studies may clarify the most effective strategies for implementing prehabilitation efforts. However, prehabilitation is intuitively important and may play a major role in the future of rehabilitation because it assigns responsibility for a successful outcome to both the patient and their health professionals.

Rehabilitation in Multimorbidity Including Cancer

Rehabilitation is usually defined in relation to one type of treatment, one disease, or in terms associated with a singular target for the intervention; however, today's patients, who often suffer from several diseases, may not receive sufficient care covering both the cancer and issues arising from other comorbid conditions. Chronic, noncommunicable health conditions form the predominant healthcare burden, and these diseases are now the main causes of morbidity and mortality in many countries. This epidemiological transition is a challenge for healthcare systems and for the rehabilitation of cancer patients. The prevalence of multimorbidity affects more than half of the global population in many countries[20] and is more prevalent among socially disadvantaged groups.[21] The literature on risk factors for multimorbidity shows that obesity across all ages is a major risk factor. Similarly, smoking is implicated in a number of diseases, a "multimorbidity group" including diabetes, cardiovascular diseases, hypertension, and cholesterol-associated disorders as well as bone, joint, and chronic obstructive lung diseases. Socioeconomic factors are major risk factors for being diagnosed with multimorbidity. This risk pattern illustrates a major target population and is an important challenge to successful rehabilitation. In addition, low health literacy, limited resources for making healthy changes in daily lifestyle, and lack of motivation are among the challenges that need to be addressed in the rehabilitation efforts of cancer survivors. Patients with multimorbidity have complex health needs, and cancer survivors with multiple chronic conditions often require complex medication regimens.[22]

The Challenge of Implementation

Despite evidence supporting rehabilitation and prehabilitation interventions, delivering them at scale is a significant challenge. Barriers include accessing a skilled workforce with programs that are integrated into cancer care, patients' motivation, symptom burden, and self-management capacity.[23] Furthermore, cultural and societal expectations also influence implementation (e.g., cancer rehabilitation is well-integrated and embedded into the healthcare system in Germany and Northern Europe, more so than elsewhere in the world).[24] These challenges, which are ubiquitous in any healthcare setting, are amplified in low-resource environments. Addressing them requires a coordinated effort at the societal, health system, and health services levels.

Professional Issues and Service Implementation

Recording and Communicating

Information obtained during the rehabilitation intervention must be included in the medical records for everyone in the healthcare system to see. Such collaboration often becomes problematic because priorities vary between sectors of the health system in every country. Uniform communication tools contribute to securing an optimal rehabilitation effort. The use of a Survivorship Passport (SCP) is crucial; this patient document includes the diagnosis and treatment provided, concurrent medications, and a short summary of functional rehabilitation interventions.

Clarify Referral Details to Community Care

Practices governing referral policies vary between countries and regions. SCP are an essential tool for exchange of information between referrals.

Legal Responsibilities

Legal responsibilities vary between countries and national legislations; these cover the responsibilities of health workers, health insurance policies, and the degree of public and/or private health programs accessible for cancer survivors.

Common Ethical Dilemmas

Competing interests can arise between the needs of the patient, caregiver, or family and the outcomes of treatments, exemplified by the long-term effects of anti-cancer treatments such as fatigue, insomnia, and depression. Gaining the support of relatives can help motivate the patient to persist with rehabilitation. Alongside this, respect for the principle of patient autonomy must prevail. Family and friends have no say in whether or not a patient participates in a rehabilitation program aside from providing transportation and support.

Low-income countries bear a disproportional burden of cancer, with estimates of 75% of cancer mortality occurring in low- and middle-income countries over the next decade.[25] When it comes to cancer rehabilitation, a scarcity of services on the ground presents a global ethical problem of disturbing inequality. This problem is more difficult to solve because of the lack of easily adaptable models of care that could inform care in low-income settings. As in other areas of rehabilitation, such as cardiac rehabilitation, the model of care delivery in low-income settings may require reliance on community health workers and peer support rather than a specialized rehabilitation workforce. The global cancer community has an imperative to forge international partnerships aimed at collaboratively designing and assessing care models that tackle this pressing challenge. As an important step in this direction, the principles of the WHO PIR are intended and designed for all resource settings.

Teams and Supervision

The teams taking care of rehabilitation may vary depending on national or local health systems. In principle, a cross-disciplinary team that uses experiences and approaches based on various disciplines may reach a level of optimal interventional effects benefitting the patient.

Implementation of Cancer Rehabilitation Programs

To improve implementation globally across all areas of health rehabilitation, the WHO established the World Rehabilitation Alliance, a global network of rehabilitation stakeholders, to undertake evidence-based advocacy focused on workforce, primary care, policy and system research, rehabilitation in emergencies, and external relations in the workstream.[26] The cancer rehabilitation package has been officially endorsed by the IPOS and the Multinational Association of Supportive Care in Cancer, making it one of the explicit priority areas contributing to this advocacy agenda.[27] These efforts can build an international momentum of advocacy and assist with sharing resources and tools. The WHO cancer package provides specific guidance on implementing context-specific rehabilitation services that address local needs.

Policy Development

At the service level, implementation efforts should ideally be informed by established implementation models or frameworks to ensure a comprehensive approach.[26,27]

Future Directions and Recommendations for Practice, Research, and Policy

- Disseminate and promote the adoption of the WHO package.
- Develop supporting tools such as implementation guides, stepped-care pathways, minimal competencies, and workforce development packages.
- Develop and evaluate models of care appropriate for low-resource settings.
- Develop a rehabilitation toolbox that accounts for multimorbidity in cancer survivors.

References

1. World Health Organization (WHO). Package of interventions for rehabilitation. Module 1. Introduction. License: CC BY-NC-SA 3.0 IGO. World Health Organization; 2023.

2. Kudre D, Chen Z, Richard A, et al. Multidisciplinary outpatient cancer rehabilitation can improve cancer patients' physical and psychosocial status: A systematic review. Curr Oncol Rep. 2020;22:1–17.

3. Stout NL, Baima J, Swisher AK, Winters-Stone KM, Welsh J. A systematic review of exercise systematic reviews in the cancer literature (2005–2017). PMR. 2017;9:S347–S384. https://pubmed.ncbi.nlm.nih.gov/35430022/

4. Shi Q, Smith TG, Michonski JD, Stein KD, Kaw C, Cleeland CS. Symptom burden in cancer survivors 1 year after diagnosis: A report from the American Cancer Society's Studies of Cancer Survivors. Cancer. 2011;117(12):2779–2790.

5. Baker P, Beesley H, Fletcher I, Ablett J, Holcombe C, Salmon P, 2016. "Getting back to normal" or "a new type of normal"? A qualitative study of patients' responses to the existential threat of cancer. Eur J Cancer Care. 2016;25(1):180–189.

6. Package of interventions for rehabilitation. Module 7. Malignant neoplasm. License: CC BY-NC-SA 3.0 IGO. World Health Organization; 2023.

7. Coderre D, Brahmbhatt P, Hunter TL, Baima J. Cancer prehabilitation in practice: The current evidence. Curr Oncol Rep. 2022;24(11):1569–1577.

8. Loeppenthin K, Oksbjerg Dalton S, Johansen C, et al. Total burden of disease in cancer patients at diagnosis: A Danish nationwide study of multimorbidity and redeemed medication. Br J Cancer. 2020;123:1033–1040. https://doi.org/10.1038/s41416-020-0950-3

9. Mitchell AJ, Chan M, Bhatti H, et al. Prevalence of depression, anxiety, and adjustment disorder in oncological, haematological, and palliative-care settings: A meta-analysis of 94 interview-based studies. Lancet Oncol. 2011;12:160–174.

10. Kjaer TK, Andersen EAW, Ursin G, et al. Cumulative incidence of second primary cancers in a large nationwide cohort of Danish cancer survivors: A population-based retrospective cohort study. Lancet Oncol. 2024;25(1):126–136. doi: 10.1016/S1470-2045(23)00538-7. Epub Dec 1, 2023. PMID: 38048803.

11. Milne HM, Wallman KE, Guilfoyle A, Gordon S, Courneya KS. Self-determination theory and physical activity among breast cancer survivors. J Sport Exercise Psychol. 2008;30:23–38. https://doi.org/10.1123/jsep.30.1.23

12. Saltbæk L, Bidstrup PE, Karlsen RV, et al. Nurse-led individualized follow-up versus regular physician-led visits after early breast cancer (MyHealth): A phase III randomized, controlled trial. J Clin Oncol. 2024;42(17):2038–2049. doi: 10.1200/JCO.23.01447. Epub Mar 18, 2024. PMID: 38498781.

13. Saltbæk L, Karlsen RV, Bidstrup PE, et al. MyHealth: Specialist nurse-led follow-up in breast cancer. A randomized controlled trial: Development and feasibility. C Acta Oncol. 2019;58(5):619–626. doi: 10.1080/0284186X.2018.1563717. Epub Jan 30, 2019. PMID: 30698065.

14. Clark J, Copsey B, Wright-Hughes A, et al. Cancer patients' needs assessment in primary care: Study protocol for a cluster randomised controlled trial (cRCT), economic evaluation and normalisation process theory evaluation of the needs assessment tool cancer (CANAssess). BMJ Open. 2022;12(5):e051394. doi: 10.1136/bmjopen-2021-051394. PMID: 35508352; PMCID: PMC9073401.

15. Signorelli, C, Hart NH, Mullen L, et al. Aligning the WHO's package of interventions for rehabilitation for cancer with the mission of IPOS: Promoting psychosocial care for all affected by cancer. J Psychosocial Oncol Res Pract. 2024;6:145–145. https://journals.lww.com/jporp/fulltext/2024/10000/aligning_the_world_health_organization_s__who_.3.aspx

16. Bandak M, Nielsen KS, Kreiberg M, et al. Smoking as a prognostic factor for survival in patients with disseminated germ cell cancer. J Natl Cancer Inst. 2023;115(6):753–756. doi: 10.1093/jnci/djad039.

17. Gao S, He Y, Jiang L, Yang J. Multimodal prehabilitation program for patients undergoing elective surgery for colorectal cancer: A scoping review. Front Oncol. 2025;15:1532624. doi: 10.3389/fonc.2025.1532624. PMID: 40386553; PMCID: PMC12082037.

18. Liao YS, Chiu HY, Huang FH, et al. Prehabilitation interventions in patients undergoing colorectal cancer surgery: A systematic review and meta-analysis. J Am Geriatr Soc. 2025:2262–2277. doi: 10.1111/jgs.19425. Epub ahead of print. PMID: 40079672.

19. White S, Mani S, Martin R, et al. Interventions provided by physiotherapists to prevent complications after major gastrointestinal cancer surgery: A systematic review and meta-analysis. Cancers (Basel). 2025;17(4):676. doi: 10.3390/cancers17040676.

20. GBD 2019 Acute and Chronic Care Collaborators. Characterising acute and chronic care needs: Insights from the Global Burden of Disease Study 2019. Nat Commun. 2025;16(1):4235. doi: 10.1038/s41467-025-56910-x. PMID: 40335470; PMCID: PMC12059133.

21. Lago-Peñas S, Rivera B, Cantarero D, Casal B, Pascual M, Blázquez-Fernández C, Reyes F. The impact of socioeconomic position on non-communicable diseases: What do we know about it? Perspect Public Health. 2021;141(3):158–176. doi: 10.1177/1757913920914952. Epub 2020 May 24. PMID: 32449467.

22. Ahmad TA, Gopal DP, Chelala C, Dayem Ullah AZ, Taylor SJ. Multimorbidity in people living with and beyond cancer: A scoping review. Am J Cancer Res. 2023;13(9):4346–4365. PMID: 37818046; PMCID: PMC10560952.

23. Raj VS, Pugh TM, Yaguda SI, Mitchell CH, Mullan SS, Garces NS. The who, what, why, when, where, and how of team-based interdisciplinary cancer rehabilitation. Semin Oncol Nurs. 2020;36(1):150974.

24. Hellbom M, Bergelt C, Bergenmar M, et al. Cancer rehabilitation: A Nordic and European perspective. Acta Oncologica. 2011;50(2):179–186.

25. Anandasabapathy S, Asirwa C, Grover S, Mungo C. Cancer burden in low-income and middle-income countries. Nat Rev Cancer. 2024;24(3):167–170. doi: 10.1038/s41568-023-00659-2.

26. Morris JH, Bernhardsson S, Bird ML, et al. Implementation in rehabilitation: A roadmap for practitioners and researchers. Disabil Rehabil. 2020;42(22):3265–3274. doi: 10.1080/09638288.2019.1587013.

27. Field B, Booth A, Ilott I, Gerrish K. Using the Knowledge to Action Framework in practice: A citation analysis and systematic review. Implement Sci. 2014;9:172. doi: 10.1186/s13012-014-0172-2.

Further Reading and Resources

ASCO. Cancer rehabilitation guidelines based on disease site or symptom. https://www.asco.org/news-initiatives/current-initiatives/cancer-care-init

iatives/prevention-survivorship/survivorship-compendium/cancer-rehab-supportive-care

ESMO. Practice guidelines. https://www.esmo.org/guidelines/esmo-clinical-practice-guidelines-supportive-and-palliative-care

Stubblefield MD, ed. *Cancer Rehabilitation: Principles and Practice*, 3rd ed. Springer, 2025.

This 90-chapter multiauthored book is an accepted classic in the field of rehabilitation.

World Health Organization (WHO). Package of interventions for rehabilitation. https://journals.lww.com/jporp/fulltext/2024/10000/aligning_the_world_health_organization_s__who_.3.aspx

Chapter 11

Health Promotion across Survivorship

Julia H. Rowland, Doris Howell, Claire Foster,
and Patricia A. Parker

Learning Objectives

After reading this chapter, the clinician will be able to:

1. Describe the drivers of the need for health promotion for cancer survivors.
2. Identify cancer screening and health behaviors that form optimal survivorship care and how to tailor these for a given patient.
3. Discuss use of the 5As and motivational interviewing (MI) to support self-management and behavior change.
4. List barriers to the engagement of cancer survivors in self-management in relation to healthy lifestyles during and after cancer treatment.
5. Identify challenges faced by healthcare providers (HCPs) in promoting screening and self-management of healthy lifestyles.

Background Evidence

Cancer and its treatment have a lasting effect on survivors' physical, psychological, social, economic, and existential health.[1] Furthermore, the cancer control continuum is not linear (prevention, detection, treatment, post-treatment/survivorship, end-of-life); instead, it is circular. Once patients are treated and cured or their disease is in remission or stable, the focus of care must circle back to prevention, early detection, and, as needed, retreatment, until that individual either dies from cancer or an unrelated cause.

🔑 Key Point
While a key goal in the past century was to improve our ability to cure or control cancer, this century will be judged by our capacity to enable people to achieve optimal health and well-being after cancer.

Screening for and early detection of cancer recurrence and new primary cancers remains a core activity of post-treatment survivorship care. Newer to this care is the addition of promoting healthy lifestyles. Health behaviors are implicated in approximately 40% of incident cancers and are a key risk factor (>75%) for developing other chronic conditions (i.e., hypertension, cardiovascular disease, diabetes).[2] Less often discussed is that these same health behaviors also influence recurrence of and survival from cancer.[3,4] Of concern is that many people do not resume or adopt healthy behaviors after a cancer diagnosis.[5] Despite evidence of benefits, cancer survivors are not uniformly counseled or supported to engage in healthy behaviors. To complicate matters, debate continues about whose job it is to promote these practices.[6,7]

As attention to cancer survivors' quality of life mounts, pressure to integrate health promotion and disease prevention into survivorship care and promote wellness is increasing. Working with health and wellness coaches and cancer peer mentors and using online programs are part of this care. Upskilling of HCPs and peers in health and wellness coaching competencies is key to improving lifestyle behaviors and health promotion. Many countries, as part of their national plans, have set standards for the integration, training, and deployment of health coaches in health systems and community care.

Key Point
To reduce unnecessary morbidity and preventable mortality, we must enhance survivors' capacity for self-management and participation in follow-up screening and health promoting activities.

Presenting Problems

Definition of Health Promotion
Health promotion and disease prevention are fundamental components of high-quality survivorship care.[8] The World Health Organization defines health promotion as "the process of enabling people to increase control over and improve their health. It moves beyond a focus on individual behavior towards a wide range of social and environmental interventions" (https://www.who.int/westernpacific/about/how-we-work/programmes/health-promotion). These goals in the context of cancer include:
- Reducing or eliminating risk for new or recurrent cancer and preventing comorbidity.
- Identifying risk for and instituting recommended interventions to minimize late effects.
- Mitigating persistent effects of cancer and its treatment.
- Optimizing clinical and self-management of comorbid conditions.
- Improving quality of life, functioning, and well-being.
- Supporting adoption and maintenance of health promoting behaviors.

Factors Driving the Need for Health Promotion

Multiple factors are driving attention to health promotion. In addition to their rise in number, cancer survivors are living longer, with more time to develop or manifest late consequences of treatment. In the United States, approximately 20% of new diagnoses are in individuals with a prior history of cancer.[9] Some of these new cancers will be iatrogenic or associated with genetic risk, but most will be secondary to aging or health behaviors (e.g., smoking, alcohol use, obesity, sedentary lifestyle, sun exposure, etc.). Additionally, most cancer survivors are older and often present with comorbid conditions,[10] which can be exacerbated by cancer treatment and warrant special management. Cancer treatment may accelerate the aging process, resulting in cumulative risks for other chronic conditions.[11] Many survivors gain weight, stop exercising, and find it challenging to engage in recommended health behaviors during and after treatment.

While important, behavior change among cancer survivors is complex. Multimodal cancer treatments often lead to clustering of late effects (e.g., cardiovascular disease, metabolic syndrome) and multimorbidities that present alongside long-term physical (e.g., reduced mobility, fatigue) and psychosocial effects (e.g., depression, low self-efficacy).[1,10] These can lead to impaired functioning, reduced capacity for self-management, and diminished motivation for health behavior change.[12] Targeting single risk behaviors (such as supervised physical activity) is increasingly viewed as inadequate, yet few HCPs are trained in health coaching or multiple behavior change.[13] Despite these hurdles, engaging in regular conversations around health promotion during and after cancer may be life altering.

Key Point

Given that survivors worry that their cancer may return and desire to learn ways to reduce their risks, we need to leverage the teachable moments to maximize uptake of health-promoting behaviors.

Investigations for Key Differential Diagnoses

Health promotion among survivors encompasses the need to assess and promote two main aspects of behavior:

- surveillance and screening for recurrent or new cancers, and
- support to engage in self-management and healthy lifestyle behaviors (see Table 11.1).

Surveillance and Screening for Cancer

Generally, screening for recurrence (surveillance) focuses on the original cancer site and common sites of new cancers secondary to cancer history (e.g., family/genetic risk, more advanced stage disease) and treatment (receipt of carcinogenic drugs and/or radiation). Screening during early recovery (years 1–2) is most intense, with follow-up visits often recommended every 3–4 months, then lengthened to every 6 months during years 3–5. By

Table 11.1 Promoting healthy behaviors after cancer

Lifestyle[a]	Screening/Early detection[b]
Alcohol	Breast cancer*
• Limit/eliminate alcohol use	• Physical breast exam
Diet	• Mammography/Ultrasound/MRI
• ↑ Fiber	Cervical cancer
• ↑ Fruits and vegetables	• HPV exposure/Vaccine
• Nuts and grains	• Pelvic exam
• ↓ Red meats	• Pap smear if appropriate
• Processed foods	Colorectal cancer
• Sugar	• FOB/stool tests
Exercise	• Colonoscopy
• ↑ Physical activity (>150 mins moderate-intensity per week, or 75 mins high-intensity)	• New blood tests
	Lung cancer
• ↓ Sitting, sedentary behavior	• CT (for increased risk groups, smoking history)
Sleep	Skin cancer /melanoma
• ↑ Meet sleep guidelines	• Full body exam
• Goal = 7–8 hours	• Monitoring of skin for moles, changes
Smoking	Prostate cancer
• Don't smoke or use other tobacco or nicotine products	• Manual exam
	• PSA
• Avoid second-hand smoke exposure	Genetic testing for increased risk:
Sun safety	BRCA1/2, Li Fraumeni syndrome, Lynch syndrome, other
• ↓ Exposure (to sun and tanning)	
• ↑ Use SPF 50 sunscreen	*Novel emerging biochemical assays to predict recurrence and/or cancer risk*
Toxins	
• Reduce workplace exposures (chemical, pesticide, radiation)	* Earlier age at screening in genetic risk families; consider MRI for dense breasts
• Safe home (avoid asbestos, lead, radon)	
Weight management	
• ↓ Obesity; Maintain healthy weight	
• BMI or weight circumference in healthy range	

[a] See Appendix A for guidelines; all behaviors listed are associated with cancer risk *except sleep.*

[b] Type and periodicity of screening recommendations for cancer survivors will vary depending on cancer treatment, age at treatment, family history, genetic profile, and other risk behaviours (e.g., smoking, alcohol use, obesity).

5 years, most survivors return to the types of cancer screening and frequency seen with non-cancer populations.

The type and frequency of screening tests for new or recurrent cancer should be tailored to cancer treatment history and personal characteristics (e.g., sex, age at treatment/currently, family history, genetic risk, screening history). Guidelines for cancer screening for the public and cancer surveillance are available across nations (see Appendix C, Survivorship Guideline Resources) and tests commonly used are included in Table 11.1.

Survivorship Care Plans

Survivorship care plans (SCPs) are an effective tool for tailoring risk-based recommendations. With the release of the IOM *Lost in Transition* report,[14] the concept of SCPs was advanced globally. They provide a roadmap for HCPs to tailor follow-up care to each person upon the end of curative cancer treatment. SCPs have two components: a treatment summary (see Table 11.2) and a follow-up care plan (see Table 11.3). Treatment summaries help identify the nature and extent of disease and treatment exposures that increase risk for late effects, which inform the type and frequency of survivorship monitoring. Follow-up care plans are intended to encompass cancer-related health promotion and disease prevention.

Ideally, SCPs are generated by the oncology team at the end of primary treatment, discussed with the survivor, and shared with other appropriate HCPs. In practice, while many survivors report receiving recommendations for the type and frequency of cancer surveillance, fewer than half receive this type of SCP. If you are following a cancer survivor, it is important to request an SCP from the oncology team or develop one if needed. SCPs are living documents to which details are added and modifications made over time.

Table 11.2 Treatment summary
1. Type of cancer (dates of diagnosis and treatment, stage, tumor characteristics)
2. Type(s) of treatment received i. Surgery (nature, extent) ii. Chemotherapy (drugs, dose, delivery) iii. Radiation (dose, port, fractionation, and schedule) iv. Immunotherapy v. Targeted therapy vi. Hormone therapy
3. Complications experienced (side effects, transfusions, recurrence/additional treatments, etc.)
4. Services used
Source: Modified from Institute of Medicine *Lost in Transition* report

Table 11.3 Follow-up care plan
1. Surveillance for recurrence or new cancer as per guidelines specific to cancer type
2. Assessment and treatment or referral for persistent effects (e.g., pain, fatigue, sexual dysfunction, functional impairment, depression, fear of cancer recurrence, employment issues)
3. Evaluation of risk for and prevention of late effects (e.g., second cancers, cardiac problems, osteoporosis); health promotion
4. Coordination of care (e.g., including frequency of visits, tests and who is performing these)
Source: Institute of Medicine *Lost in Transition* report.

> **Box 11.1 Screening and Assessment**
>
> Screening and assessment as part of routine clinical care should determine
> 1. Current physical and mental health status and health behaviors, taking into account other conditions and their impacts on daily life
> 2. Risk factors that may act as barriers to engaging with health promotion
> 3. Iatrogenic late effects that might impact engagement with health behaviors (e.g., anthracycline use and cardiovascular disease; chest irradiation and subsequent breast cancer risk)
> 4. Nature of support required so that care and support can be tailored accordingly

Beyond surveillance for recurrence, as survivors age, HCPs need to recommend screening for other cancers (e.g., prostate, colorectal, lung cancer).

Healthy Lifestyle Behaviors

HCPs also need to evaluate survivors' current health behaviors and provide guidance on how to improve these (see Table 11.1). There is no standard form for lifestyle assessment. However, questions about these behaviors should be part of regular follow-up visits including questions that enable HCPs to ascertain if the patient is meeting the desired levels of each behavior (see Box 11.1).

Addressing Barriers to Behavior Change

After ascertaining lifestyle behaviors there should also be assessment of barriers to engaging in screening and health promotion. This allows consideration of the impact on survivors of aging, sociodemographic factors, comorbid conditions, late effects, mental health concerns, low self-efficacy, and low social support.[15] Barriers to behavior change may be present on multiple levels (see Table 11.4). For example, with respect to cancer screening and surveillance, delays and/or missed appointments may be due to overwhelming fear of test results. Identifying anxiety and strategies to cope with it, including referral for counseling as needed, is important (see Chapter 3). Helping survivors prioritize healthy behaviors and ways to incorporate these practices into their daily routine is important.

Assessments that build a picture of the "whole person" enable HCPs to understand the individual's unique barriers to engaging in health promotion. An appreciation of the contribution of these domains to facilitating or impeding change can increase success in supporting change.

🔍 Key Point

It is important to note that HCPs often underestimate the positive impact their recommendation for and support of a particular practice has on their patients' subsequent behavior.

Table 11.4 Barriers to health behavior change

1. **Intrapersonal:** Believe at low risk for recurrence or invulnerability; low self-efficacy to engage in behavior change; low motivation to change

2. **Interpersonal:** Low/no support to engage in healthy behaviors; limited financial resources

3. **Organizational:** Low/no support for change from oncology or primary care providers and settings

4. **Community:** Low/no neighborhood resources (e.g., limited walkable spaces, health facilities)

5. **Sociocultural:** Low/no support from neighbors, community, cultural groups for adoption/practice of healthy behaviours

6. **Time:** Competing demands from family, work, school, social/leisure time; problems managing time

Modeled after Bronfenbrenner's work, *Ecological Systems Theory.* Jessica Kingsley; 1992.

Clinical Management

Championing Health Promotion: Whose Job Is It?

The debate over who should provide survivorship care and how this care is delivered is long-standing. Central professionals are oncology and primary care providers (PCPs). Arguably, those who treat cancer should hold some responsibility for the outcomes of patients in their care, but, as patients live longer, this becomes an impossible task since newly diagnosed patients need to be seen and treated. Furthermore, oncology, a specialty service, is not well designed to provide whole-person medical care (e.g., monitor diabetes, ensure delivery of appropriate vaccines, promote healthy lifestyle). These aspects of health are generally the purview of primary care. Yet PCPs report anxiety around delivering follow-up care to cancer survivors in their practice, especially about cancer surveillance, and often refer these patients back to their oncologists.[6,7] Many PCPs have minimal training in cancer survivorship care and feel ill-equipped to manage and support the unique needs of survivors in their practice.[16]

In some countries, such as in the United Kingdom's National Health Service (NHS), follow-up care is stratified according to risks, with rapid access to oncology support specified in pathways of care if patients or HCPs are concerned about cancer recurrence. Patients who are at low risk of recurrence and have low needs are stratified to self-managed follow-up. Patients with more complex needs or at higher risk of recurrence have follow-up directed by oncology teams. (https://www.longtermplan.nhs.uk/). Shared care models may be a solution well suited for high- risk survivors, whereas primary care-led, nurse-led, or patient-led/-supported self-management models are appropriate for low-risk survivors and hold promise for championing health promotion.[17]

🔍 Key Point

In the end, more important than by whom this care is delivered is that a designated individual (or individuals) is responsible for championing this aspect of survivors' health.

Raising Awareness and Understanding

Arguably, the most critical step to supporting cancer survivors with engagement in health promotion and disease prevention is to raise awareness of how their behavior can prevent or mitigate risk for adverse health outcomes. Developing and disseminating education and communication strategies can shift attitudes toward lifestyle behavior change for both HCPs and cancer survivors.

Talking to patients around the time of diagnosis about their health behaviors and what they can do to improve their health and wellness reinforces the expectation that they will be a survivor. These conversations provide a positive, future-focused message that there is something they can do at a time when things can feel uncertain. It is a way to identify areas in which they *do* have control and can, through self-management, play an active role in managing their illness. Conversations about health promotion should continue during treatment and, importantly, be revisited at transition to follow-up care and ongoing.

HCPs play a key role in supporting long-term health promotion by encouraging healthy behaviors; being aware of available support such as nutrition, physical activity, and smoking cessation programs; monitoring long-term effects of cancer and treatment; and identifying appropriate interventions. This means being up to date with current health behavior guidelines for cancer survivors and available resources for HCP and patient education[8] (see Appendix D for training resources).

Supporting Behavior Change

Fostering Self-Management

To be successful, support for self-management and behavior change needs to involve a partnership between HCPs and cancer survivors that identifies who is responsible for what, as part of follow-up care. Emerging evidence supports the effectiveness of self-management support (SMS) and/or health and wellness coaching in promoting health behavior change.[17] SMS is a core element of survivorship models of care delivered in partnership with survivors and HCPs or trained peers. Effective SMS requires evidence-based, structured programs and health care coaching to support survivors to gain confidence and capacity to build self-management skills. These skills include problem-solving, decision-making, self-monitoring, and goals to facilitate the uptake of healthy lifestyle behaviors.[24]

Promoting Healthy Lifestyle Behavior Change

SMS is more than patient education. Critically, approaches using passive dissemination of information are ineffectual: instead, behavior change methods such as the 5As framework (assess, advise, agree, assist, arrange) and MI are recommended[18,19] (see Box 11.2).

A "stepped model" for supporting the uptake of self-management strategies and healthy lifestyle behavior change may be needed to optimize resources. The first step on a model such as the 5As framework could be initiated as a universal approach for behavior change coaching within routine HCP practices, with more intensive interventions added based on need, health risks, and complexity of behavior change.[19]

Box 11.2 Abbreviated 5As Coaching for Behavior Change

Establish rapport: Move from telling what to do and shaming to leverage strengths.

Assess: At pre-visit behavioral assessment, invite people to talk about health concerns and collaboratively set priorities for lifestyle change and desired outcomes (i.e., weight loss, etc.).

Advise: Tailor to the individual, condition(s), capacity, advice/options for change with permission.

Agree: Assess readiness, scale importance of behavior change (NRS 0–10 scale) (explore the why), identify preferred actions/options for change and commitment to reduce resistance.

Assist:- Guide SMART (specific, measurable, attainable, realistic/relevant, time bound) goals and action plan. Scale level of confidence (0 = no confidence to 10 = high confidence; should be ≥7), set self-monitoring plan (e.g., use digital tracking device for physical activity).

Arrange: Appropriate assistance (self-help behavior change materials) and referrals for additional support (e.g., smoking cessation clinic, exercise specialist, nutritionist). Importantly: follow up.

The 5As framework is recommended as a universal structured approach with established efficacy for smoking cessation, weight and obesity management, alcohol and substance misuse, improving physical activity and reducing sedentary behavior, and healthy eating. The 5As coaching process, based on Prochaska's transtheoretical model of change,[20] is championed for HCPs given its simplicity and utility for use in brief clinical encounters (i.e., 10–15 minutes). Embedded within the 5As are strategies key to motivating behavior change and building self-efficacy in taking health actions (i.e., goal setting and action planning, teach-back, problem-solving barriers to action, rulers for scaling importance of behavior, readiness, and confidence).

Training initiatives support PCPs in the application of the 5As of behavior change.[21] Toolkits and specific examples showing the application of the 5As behavior change counseling in smoking cessation, healthy eating, and obesity management have been developed (see Appendix E, Resources for Training).

Motivational Interviewing

Many survivors will require more intensive behavior change counseling using techniques such as MI, defined as a "directive, client-centered counselling style for eliciting behavior change by helping clients to explore and resolve ambivalence to behavior change."[22] The core processes of MI behavior change counseling are shown in Box 11.3 and include many techniques and skills to effect and sustain change.

There is robust evidence for the efficacy of MI to reduce ambivalence and resistance to health behavior change,[22,23] but specific training in MI is required, and MI-adherent coaching is key to improving outcomes. Brief MI techniques can be incorporated into the 5As coaching process and used in routine practice.

Box 11.3 Core Processes of Motivational Interviewing

- **Engagement:** Develop a therapeutic working alliance using person-centered communication skills (OARS = open-ended questions, affirmations, reflections, summaries)
- **Focusing:** Identify targeted behavior the patient is ready and able to change
- **Evoking:** Talk about change and intrinsic motivation or "why change"
- **Planning:** Develop specific plan for health behavior change (goals and actions)

🔍 Key Point

Consideration should be given to integration of health coaching in survivorship services and cancer community and peer support organizations.

Case Study

Angela is a 36-year-old woman, newly married, and she has a new PCP. She was diagnosed with stage II, triple negative breast cancer at age 28 and treated with mastectomy without reconstruction, plus six rounds of chemotherapy with paclitaxel and doxorubicin; she has been disease-free ever since and is no longer followed by her treating oncologist. Her menses, which became irregular during chemotherapy, are mostly regular now. She and her husband hope to start a family right away.

She is moderately overweight, being largely sedentary and working long hours as a partner at a law firm. Her physical exam is unremarkable except for a well-healed right mastectomy scar; all her blood work comes back normal. She is mildly hypertensive (140/88) and remains so on re-examination. She has a family history of cancer, both breast and non-breast. No genetic testing was done when she was diagnosed. Her concerns are being able to conceive, anxiety about leaving her oncologist, and self-consciousness about being overweight.

She was not given an SCP by her oncologist, so together she and the PCP draft one. With her consent, the PCP plans to contact her former oncologist for more information on her cancer care. Based on the information shared, her PCP recommends (1) continuing regular annual mammographic screening of her left breast as recommended by her oncologist; (2) referral to a genetic counselor to see if the pattern of cancer occurrence in her family warrants testing for susceptibility genes and to inform the care of potential offspring; (3) referral to a cardiologist (cardio-oncologist if available) based on her hypertension and exposure to doxorubicin, which is cardiotoxic at higher doses; and (4) referral to a fertility specialist to evaluate her current hormonal status. Her PCP can reassure her that, being more than 5 years post-diagnosis, published data do not indicate increased problems with conceiving or childbearing and are like those of similarly aged women in the general population. In addition, they discuss ways to lose weight and include more physical activity in her daily routine. She states that exercise is most important to her right now, and she is not ready to talk about her weight. Their conversation includes eliciting information on what exercise she has previously enjoyed (dance classes at her gym, cycling) and any barriers (time, gym access). Her PCP offers to refer her to a personal trainer. To meet her goals, she will need to prioritize exercise. They schedule a 3-month follow-up to review progress and correct course as needed.

Professional Issues and Service Implementation

To date, health promotion and disease prevention as essential components of survivorship care have not been fully operationalized, and no entity in the healthcare system has claimed major responsibility for tackling this aspect of survivors' care. Beyond this fundamental barrier to care, HCPs face several other challenges and barriers to supporting health promotion for cancer survivors.

Insufficient Number of Providers

The biggest barrier is insufficient numbers of HCPs to provide survivorship care (e.g., oncologists, PCPs, nurse practitioners). Therefore, teams need to be expanded to meet this need (e.g., community health workers, peer mentors/coaches), and the proactive initiation of survivors in self-management and training is critical to the scaling up of health promotion efforts.

Training

The American Society of Clinical Oncology has published guidelines for what should be encompassed in survivorship education.[8] Survivorship education for nurses is growing as more nurses take the lead in survivors' care.[24] PCPs play a vital role in prevention, early intervention, and management of lifestyle-related diseases. The United Kingdom has targeted the training of PCPs in the requisite knowledge and skills for effective counseling in lifestyle behavior change (https://www.england.nhs.uk/personalisedcare). The American College of Preventive Medicine has also taken a lead role in setting out the core competencies for lifestyle behavior change and targeting PCPs in this regard.

Importantly, HCPs do not need to be expert in all aspects of health promotion for survivors. Advances in artificial intelligence (AI) have created new avenues for education and support. Currently, programs are being developed and evaluated with AI-based personalized health coaches.

Of note, it is not always necessary to provide in-depth health coaching because many survivors are motivated to take action to improve their health behaviors.[25]

Communication and Coordination of Care

A further challenge is the critical need to improve communication and coordination of care among oncology teams, PCPs, and patients and caregivers.[26,27] Clear delineation of roles and responsibilities for recommending and overseeing different aspects of care following a cancer diagnosis is essential.

Electronic health records can facilitate communication among HCPs and between patients and HCPs. Patient portals can be used to communicate about health promotion plans. At the same time, the use of digital formats serves to provide individual support and counseling to survivors, thus reducing the burden of clinician delivery.[28]

Cultural Issues

Cultural factors affect many aspects of survivorship care including health promotion. Diet and exercise patterns and health resources vary across cultures and need to be elicited and understood when making recommendations. Cultural beliefs and practices may affect how individuals participate in health promotion. For example, an integrative review found that many aspects of culture including values, beliefs, social norms, religiosity, and sex roles influence engagement in various self-management behaviors including eating a healthy diet, physical activity, and managing stress.[29]

Time and Cost

Another key consideration is the financial aspect of this care. Additionally, HCPs are attending to multiple aspects of care during cancer survivorship and may not have sufficient time to address health promotion during appointments.

Barriers to providing comprehensive survivorship care occur at multiple levels (patient, provider, system, societal, governmental/health policy, advocacy), requiring time, investment, and innovative solutions. At the same time, pressure to address the well-being of survivors is creating exciting opportunities for growth and change by

- Encouraging patient self-management and investment in well-being
- Empowering HCPs to offer comprehensive, person-centered care
- Engaging HCPs to better understand and find ways to
  - o reduce the late effects of cancer with novel and targeted therapies;
  - o develop interventions to minimize future health risks
- Broadening our understanding of how best to help people adopt and maintain healthy behaviors
- Expanding knowledge to promote the well-being of those with and without cancer

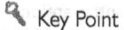 Key Point

Investments in this aspect of survivors' care today holds the promise of long-term benefit to reduce the global burden of cancer tomorrow.

References

1. Emery J, Butow P, Lai-Kwon J, et al. Management of common clinical problems experienced by survivors of cancer. Lancet. 2022;399(10334):1537–1550. doi: 10.1016/S0140-6736(22)00242-2. PMID: 35430021.

2. Islami F, Marlow EC, Thomson B, et al. Proportion and number of cancer cases and deaths attributable to potentially modifiable risk factors in the United States, 2019. CA Cancer J Clin. 2024;74(5):405–432. doi: 10.3322/caac.21858. PMID: 38990124.

3. Bian Z, Zhang R, Yuan S, et al. Healthy lifestyle and cancer survival: A multinational cohort study. Int J Cancer. 2024;154(10):1709–1718. doi: 10.1002/ijc.34846. PMID: 38230569.

4. Matta K, Viallon V, Botteri E, et al. Healthy lifestyle change and all-cause and cancer mortality in the European Prospective Investigation into Cancer and Nutrition cohort. BMC Med. 2024;22(1):210. doi: 10.1186/s12916-024-03362-7. PMID: 38807179.

5. Gregory K, Zhao L, Felder TM, et al. Prevalence of health behaviors among cancer survivors in the United States. J Cancer Surviv. 2024;18(3):1042–1050. doi: 10.1007/s11764-023-01347-8. PMID: 36933085.

6. Vos JAM, Wollersheim BM, Cooke A, et al. Primary care physicians' knowledge and confidence in providing cancer survivorship care: A systematic review. J Cancer Surviv. 2024;18(5):1557–1573. doi: 10.1007/s11764-023-01397-y. PMID: 37171716.

7. Fauer AJ, Ganz PA, Brauer ER. A mixed method study of medical oncologists' perceived barriers and motivators to addressing long-term effects in breast cancer survivors. Breast Cancer Res Treat. 2022;194(3):699–707. doi: 10.1007/s10549-022-06657-6. PMID: 35767127.

8. Shapiro CL, Jacobsen PB, Henderson T, et al. ReCAP: ASCO core curriculum for cancer survivorship education. J Oncol Pract. 2016;12(2):145, e108–117. doi: 10.1200/JOP.2015.009449. PMID: 26813926.

9. Forjaz G, Howlader N, Scoppa S, et al. Impact of including second and later cancers in cause-specific survival estimates using population-based registry data. Cancer. 2022;128(3):547–557. doi: 10.1002/cncr.33940. PMID: 34623641.

10. Jiang C, Deng L, Karr MA, et al. Chronic comorbid conditions among adult cancer survivors in the United States: Results from the National Health Interview Survey, 2002–2018. Cancer. 2022;128(4):828–838. doi: 10.1002/cncr.33981. PMID: 34706057.

11. Guida JL, Ahles TA, Belsky D, et al. Measuring aging and identifying aging phenotypes in cancer survivors. J Natl Cancer Inst. 2019;111(12):1245–1254. doi: 10.1093/jnci/djz136. PMID: 31321426.

12. Hoedjes M, Nijman I, Hinnen C. Psychosocial determinants of lifestyle change after a cancer diagnosis: A systematic review of the literature. Cancers. 2022;14(8):2026. doi: 10.3390/cancers14082026. PMID: 35454932.

13. Silva CC, Presseau J, van Allen Z, et al. Effectiveness of interventions for changing more than one behavior at a time to manage chronic conditions: A systematic review and meta-analysis. Ann Behav Med. 2024;23:58(6):432–444. doi: 10.1093/abm/kaae021. PMID: 3872198.

14. Institute of Medicine and National Research Council. (2006). *From Cancer Patient to Cancer Survivor: Lost in Transition*. National Academies Press. https://doi.org/10.17226/11468. ISBN: 978-0-309-09595-2

15. Foster C, Haviland J, Winter J, et al. Pre-surgery depression and confidence to manage problems predict recovery trajectories of health and wellbeing in the first two years following colorectal cancer: Results from the CREW cohort study. PLoS One. 2016;11(5):e0155434. doi: 10.1371/journal.pone.0155434. PMID: 27171174.

16. Crabtree BF, Miller WL, Howard J, et al. Cancer survivorship care roles for primary care physicians. Ann Fam Med. 2020;18(3):202–209. doi: 10.1370/afm.2498. PMID: 32393555.

17. Jefford M, Howell D, Li Q, et al. Improved models of care for cancer survivors. Lancet. 2022;399(10334):1551–1560. doi: 10.1016/S0140-6736(22)00306-3. PMID: 35430022.

18. Howell D, Mayer DK, Fielding R, et al.; Global Partners for Self-Management in Cancer. Management of cancer and health after the clinic visit: A call to action for self-management in cancer care. J Natl Cancer Inst. 2021;4113(5):523–531. doi: 10.1093/jnci/djaa083. PMID: 32525530.

19. Glasgow RE, Emont S, Miller DC. Assessing delivery of the five 'As' for patient-centered counseling. Health Promot Int. 2006;21(3):245–255. doi: 10.1093/heapro/dal017. PMID: 16751630.

20. Prochaska JO, Velicer WF, Redding C, et al. Stage-based expert systems to guide a population of primary care patients to quit smoking, eat healthier, prevent skin cancer, and receive regular mammograms. Prev Med. 2005;41(2):406–416. doi: 10.1016/j.ypmed.2004.09.050. PMID: 15896835.

21. Frates B, Ortega HA, Freeman KJ, et al. Lifestyle medicine in medical education: Maximizing impact. Mayo Clin Proc Innov Qual Outcomes. 2024;8(5):451–474. doi: 10.1016/j.mayocpiqo.2024.07.003. PMID: 39263429.

22. Shaw DS, Wilson MN. Taking a motivational interviewing approach to prevention science: Progress and extensions. Prev Sci. 2021;22(6):826–830. doi: 10.1007/s11121-021-01269-w. PMID: 34173134.

23. Harkin K, Apostolopoulos V, Tangalakis K, et al. The impact of motivational interviewing on behavioural change and health outcomes in cancer patients and survivors. A systematic review and meta-analysis. Maturitas. 2023;170:9–21. doi: 10.1016/j.maturitas.2023.01.004. PMID: 36736204.

24. Grant M, McCabe M, Economou D. Nurse education and survivorship: Building the specialty through training and program development. Clin J Oncol Nurs. 2017;21(4):454–459. doi: 10.1188/17.CJON.454-459. PMID: 28738038.

25. Grimmett C, Corbett T, Brunet J, et al. Systematic review and meta-analysis of maintenance of physical activity behaviour change in cancer survivors. Int J Behav Nutr Phys Act. 2019;16(1):37. doi: 10.1186/s12966-019-0787-4. PMID: 31029140.

26. Lisy K, Kent J, Piper A, Jefford M. Facilitators and barriers to shared primary and specialist cancer care: A systematic review. Support Care Cancer. 2021;29:85–96. doi: 10.1007/s00520-020-05624-5. PMID: 32803729.

27. Parker PA, Banerjee SC, Matasar MJ, et al. Efficacy of a survivorship-focused consultation versus a time-controlled rehabilitation consultation in patients with lymphoma: A cluster randomized controlled trial. Cancer. 2018;124(23):4567–4576. doi: 10.1002/cncr.31767. PMID: 30335188.

28. Roberts AL, Fisher A, Smith L et al. Digital health behaviour change interventions targeting physical activity and diet in cancer survivors: A systematic review and meta-analysis. J Cancer Surviv. 2017;11(6):704–719. doi: 10.1007/s11764-017-0632-1. PMID: 28779220.

29. Yeom JW, Yeom IS, Park HY, Lim SH. Cultural factors affecting the self-care of cancer survivors: An integrative review. Eur J Oncol Nurs. 2022;59:102165. doi: 10.1016/j.ejon.2022.102165. PMID: 35777220.

Further Reading

Chan RJ, Crawford-Williams F, Crichton M, et al. Effectiveness and implementation of models of cancer survivorship care: An overview of systematic reviews. J Cancer Surviv. 2023;17(1):197–221. doi: 10.1007/s11764-021-01128-1. PMID: PMID: 34786652.

Halpern M, Mollica MA, Han PKJ, Tonorezos ES. Myths and presumptions about cancer survivorship. J Clin Oncol. 2024;42(2):134–139. doi: 10.1200/JCO.23.00631. Epub 2023 Nov 16. PMID: PMID: 37972343; PMCID: PMC10824378.

Institute of Medicine and National Research Council. (2006). *From Cancer Patient to Cancer Survivor: Lost in Transition.* National Academies Press. https://doi.org/10.17226/11468. ISBN: 978-0-309-09595-2

Mollica MA, McWhirter G, Tonorezos E, et al.; National Cancer Survivorship Standards Subject Matter Expert Group. Developing national cancer survivorship standards to inform quality of care in the United States using a consensus approach. J Cancer Surviv. 2024;18(4):1190–1199. doi: 10.1007/s11764-024-01602-6. Erratum in: J Cancer Surviv. 2024 Aug;18(4):1200. doi: 10.1007/s11764-024-01618-y. PMID: 38739299; PMCID: PMC11324674. May 13. doi: 10.1007/s11764-024-01602-6. Erratum in: J Cancer Surviv. 2024 Jun 15. doi: 10.1007/s11764-024-01618-y. PMID: 38739299.

Salathiel E, Passmore J. (2021). *Does Health Coaching Work: A Critical Review of the Evidence of Coaching in Health Care Systems.* Henley Business School; 2021. ISBN 978-1-912473-30-4.

Appendix A

Measurement Tools for Differential Work-Related Issues

- **Work Ability Index (WAI):** Measures current work ability compared to lifetime best, work demands, health status, and mental resources.
  Ilmarinen J. The Work Ability Index (WAI). Occup Med. 2007;57(2):160. https://doi.org/10.1093/occmed/kqm008
- **Work Role Functioning Questionnaire (WRFQ):** Assesses perceived work functioning across physical, social, emotional, and cognitive domains.
  Amick BC, Lerner D, Rogers WH, Rooney T, Katz JN. A review of health-related work outcome measures and their uses, and recommended measures. Spine 2000;25:3152.
- **The "Readiness for Return to Work" (RRTW) questionnaire:** Facilitates intervention development tailored to cancer survivors' needs, related to the return to work stage.
  Franche RL, Corbière M, Lee H, Breslin FC, Hepburn CG. The Readiness for Return-To-Work (RRTW) scale: Development and validation of a self-report staging scale in lost-time claimants with musculoskeletal disorders. J Occup Rehabil. 2007;17(3):450–472. doi: 10.1007/s10926-007-9097-9. Epub 2007 Aug 15. PMID: 17701326.
- **Work Limitations Questionnaire (WLQ):** Assesses limitations in performing job demands due to health problems.
  Lerner D, Amick BC 3rd, Rogers WH, Malspeis S, Bungay K, Cynn D. The Work Limitations Questionnaire. Med Care. 2001;39(1):72–85. doi: 10.1097/00005650-200101000-00009. PMID: 11176545.
- **Return-to-Work Self-Efficacy Scale (RTW-SE):** Measures confidence in ability to return to work following health issues.
  Lagerveld SE, Blonk WB, Brenninkmeijer V, Schaufeli WB. Return to work among employees with mental health problems: Development and validation of a self-efficacy questionnaire. Work Stress. 2010;24(4):359–375.
- **Utrecht Work Engagement Scale (UWES):** Measures work engagement, an important factor for sustained work ability.
  Schaufeli W, Bakker A. UWES Utrecht Work Engagement Scale. Preliminary Manual [Version 1, November 2003]. Utrecht University: Occupational Health Psychology Unit; 2003.

- **Multidimensional Fatigue Inventory (MFI):** Measures fatigue severity, including general, physical, and mental fatigue.

  Smets EM, Garssen B, Bonke B, De Haes JC. The Multi-dimensional Fatigue Inventory (MFI) psychometric qualities of an instrument to assess fatigue. J Psychosom Res. 1995;39:315–325.

- **Cancer Worry Scale (CWS):** Assesses worries about developing cancer or developing cancer again and the impact of these concerns on daily functioning.

  Custers JAE, Van Den Berg SW, Van Laarhoven HWM, Bleiker EMA, Gielissen MFM, Prins JB. The Cancer Worry Scale: Detecting fear of recurrence in breast cancer survivors. Cancer Nurs. 2014.;37(1):E44–50. doi: 10.1097/NCC.0b013e3182813a17. PMID: 23448956.

- **European Organization for Research and Treatment for Cancer Quality of Life Questionnaire (EORTC QLQ C30):** Includes a specific item measuring financial difficulties due to disease or treatment.

  Aaronson NK, Ahmedzai S, Bergman B, et al. The European Organization for Research and Treatment of Cancer QLQ-C30: A quality-of-life instrument for use in international clinical trials in oncology. JNCI 1993;85(5):365–376.

- **Subjective Financial Distress Questionnaire (SFDQ):** Measures perceived financial stress and its psychological impact on individuals, focusing on their subjective experience of financial strain.

  Dar MA, Chauhan R, Murti K, Trivedi V and Dhingra S. Development and validation of Subjective Financial Distress Questionnaire (SFDQ): A patient reported outcome measure for assessment of financial toxicity among radiation oncology patients. Front Oncol. 2022;11:819313. doi: 10.3389/fonc.2021.819313.

- **Comprehensive Score for Financial Toxicity Instrument (COST):** Measures the financial burden and distress experienced by patients as a result of medical treatment costs.

  de Souza JA, Yap BJ, Wroblewski K, et al. Measuring financial toxicity as a clinically relevant patient-reported outcome: The validation of the COmprehensive Score for financial Toxicity (COST). Cancer. 2017;123(3):476–484. doi: 10.1002/cncr.30369. Epub 2016 Oct 7. PMID: 27716900; PMCID: PMC5298039.

Appendix B

AYA Additional Screening Tools

Tools for Adolescents and Young Adults

- **Brief Symptom Inventory (BSI)-18**
  https://www.pearsonassessments.com/store/usassessments/en/Store/Professional-Assessments/Personality-%26-Biopsychosocial/Brief-Symptom-Inventory-18/p/100000638.html

- **Posttraumatic Stress Response Diagnostic Scale (PDS)**
  McCarthy S. Post-Traumatic Stress Diagnostic Scale (PDS). Occup Med. 2008;58(5):379. https://doi.org/10.1093/occmed/kqn062.

- **General Health Questionnaire (GHQ)**
  https://www.gl-assessment.co.uk/products/general-health-questionnaire-ghq/

- **Cancer Worry Scale**
  Custers JAE, Kwakkenbos L, van de Wal M, Prins JB, Thewes B. Re-validation and screening capacity of the 6-item version of the Cancer Worry Scale. Psycho-Oncology. 2018;27:2609–2615. https://doi.org/10.1002/pon.4782

- **Fear of Cancer Recurrence Inventory (FCRI)**
  Smith AB, Costa D, Galica J, et al. Spotlight on the Fear of Cancer Recurrence Inventory (FCRI). Psychol Res Behav Manag. 202021;13:1257–1268. doi: 10.2147/PRBM.S231577. PMID: 33376421; PMCID: PMC7762428.

- **Pediatric Quality of Life Inventory (PedsQL)**
  Varni JW, Seid M, Kurtin PS. PedsQL 4.0: Reliability and validity of the Pediatric Quality of Life Inventory version 4.0 generic core scales in healthy and patient populations. Med Care. 2001;39(8):800–812. doi: 10.1097/00005650-200108000-00006. PMID: 11468499.6.

- **Impact of Cancer-Childhood Survivors (IOC-CS)**
  Zebrack BJ, et al. Psychometric evaluation of the Impact of Cancer (IOC-CS) scale for young adult survivors of childhood cancer. Qual Life Res. 2010;19(2):207–218. https://pmc.ncbi.nlm.nih.gov/articles/PMC2906664/

Tools for AYA Parents and Families

Parent and Family

- **The Psychosocial Assessment Tool (PAT 3.0):** A standardized parent self-report of psychosocial risk in families of children with cancer assessing family functioning, social support, acute stress, anxiety, child behavior, and sibling's problems.

https://pubmed.ncbi.nlm.nih.gov/29509908/

• **Distress Thermometer for Parents (DT-P):** A standardized tool that generates a 1–10 unidimensional rating of distress in parents of children with chronic illness as a general checklist measure addressing emotional, physical, practical, social, and spiritual concerns.

https://www.sciencedirect.com/science/article/pii/S0022347613007245

Patient or Caregiver (Proxy)

• **PedsQL General Core Scales:** Child and parent proxy measures physical, emotional, social, and school functioning.

Pedsql.org

• **PROMIS Pediatric Mental Health Measures:** Child and parent proxy measures of global health (physical and mental health) as well as specific domains: emotional distress, anxiety, depression, anger, positive affect).

HealthMeasures.net

• **PROMIS Adult Mental Health Measures:** Global health (physical and mental health) as well as specific domains: emotional distress, anxiety, depression, anger, positive affect).

HealthMeasures.net

• **NIH Toolbox Emotion Measures (Child and Parent Proxy):** Neuro-behavioral measures of cognitive and emotional functioning (negative affect, psychological wellbeing, stress and self-efficacy, social relationships).

HealthMeasures.net

• **Checking IN:** A pediatric and proxy electronic self-report distress screening tool of psychosocial symptoms that can interfere with quality of life. Generates an immediate summary report for clinical management.

https://www.cancersupportcommunity.org/checking-in

• **Survivors 12–17 -- Beck Youth Scales Anxiety, Depression.**

https://www.pearsonclinical.co.uk/Psychology/ChildMentalHealth/ChildMentalHealth/BeckYouthInventories-SecondEditionForChildrenand Adolescents(BYI-II)/BeckYouthInventories-SecondEditionForChildrenand Adolescents(BYI-II).aspx

• **Childhood Cancer Survivors 18 or Older -- BSI-18.**

https://www.pearsonassessments.com/store/usassessments/en/Store/Professional-Assessments/Personality-%26-Biopsychosocial/Brief-Symptom-Inventory-18/p/100000638.html

• **PHQ-9:**

https://www.med.umich.edu/1info/FHP/practiceguides/depress/phq-9.pdf

• **PHQ-2:**

https://brightfutures.aap.org/Bright%20Futures%20Documents/PHQ-2%20Instructions%20for%20Use.pdf

- **Impact of Cancer-Childhood Survivors (IOC-CS):**
  https://pmc.ncbi.nlm.nih.gov/articles/PMC2906664/
- **Childhood Cancer Survivor Study (CCSS) – Needs Assessment Questionnaire (CCSS-NAQ):**
  https://pmc.ncbi.nlm.nih.gov/articles/PMC5341614/
- **EORTC: Adolescent and young adult questionnaire:**
  https://qol.eortc.org/questionnaire/aya/
- **EORTC: Survivorship Questionnaire:**
  https://qol.eortc.org/questionnaire/surv100/

Tools for Neuropsychological Assessment

Examples of monitoring tools that can be used for screening. All are available at https://ascopubs.org/doi/10.1200/JCO.20.02444

- **Vanderbilt Assessment Scale:** ADHD, age range 6–12 years.
- **Colorado Learning Differences Questionnaire:** Learning difficulties, parent reported.
- **Bayley Scales of Infant Development Screening Test-III/IV:** Age range 16 days to 42 months
- **Reynolds Intellectual Screening Test-2:** General intelligence screening, 3–94 years.
- **Wechsler Scales:** Global cognitive functioning, age range 16–90 years.
- **Delis-Kaplan Executive Function System:** Verbal fluency, color–word, interference, and trail-making test; tests executive function, age range 8–89 years.

Resources for Post-Treatment Transition and AYA Survivorship Care

- **Health Links from COG, LTFU guidelines**
  https://www.gottransition.org/
- **Passport to Care**
  https://passportforcare.org/
- **LTFU guidelines**
  Poplack DG, Fordis M, Landier W, et al. Childhood cancer survivor care: Development of the Passport for Care. Nat Rev Clin Oncol. 2014;11(12):740–750. doi: 10.1038/nrclinonc.2014.175 https://www.ncbi.nlm.nih.gov/pmc/articles/PMC5142740/
- **PanCare Survivorship Passport (PanCareSurPass)**
  https://www.survivorshippassport.org/
- **Transition to adult care**
  https://www.gottransition.org/

- **National Cancer Institute: Care for Childhood Cancer Survivors**
  https://www.cancer.gov/about-cancer/coping/survivorship/child-care
- **COG Survivorship Guidelines**
  http://www.survivorshipguidelines.org/
- **Finding and paying for healthcare:** In English, Spanish, Chinese traditional (TC), and Chinese simplified SC)
- **Introduction to long-term follow-up:** In English, Spanish, Chinese traditional (TC), and Chinese simplified SC)
- **American Society of Clinical Oncology (ASCO) – Cancer in Young Adults**
  https://www.cancer.net/navigating-cancer-care/young-adults-and-teenagers
- **CanTeen**
  https://www.canteen.org.au/
- **Children's Oncology Group, Coping with Cancer**
  https://childrensoncologygroup.org/index.php/81-coping-with-cancer
- **LIVESTRONG Adolescents and Young Adults**
  https://www.livestrong.org/we-can-help/young-adults
- **Teenage Cancer Trust**
  https://www.teenagecancertrust.org/about-us
- **Stupid Cancer**
  https://stupidcancer.org/
- **Ulman Foundation**
  https://ulmanfoundation.org/

Interventions for AYA Survivorship Care

Examples of interventions with empirical support:

Cognitive Behavior Therapy (CBT): Parent or Child

- **Cognitive Behavior Group Intervention**
  https://pubmed.ncbi.nlm.nih.gov/36537338/
- **Cognitive Behavior Group Intervention:** Parents.
  https://pubmed.ncbi.nlm.nih.gov/36537338/
- **Bright IDEAS Problem Solving Skills therapy (PSST):** Available in English and Spanish.
  https://rtips.cancer.gov/rtips/programDetails.do?programId=546012
  https://open.learnbrightideas.org/
- **Surviving Cancer Competently Intervention Program (SCCIP):** Parent.
  https://rtips.cancer.gov/rtips/programDetails.do?programId=102875

- **Acceptance and Commitment Therapy**
  https://contextualscience.org/act
- **Recapture Life**
  https://pubmed.ncbi.nlm.nih.gov/34070134/

Survivorship Guideline Resources

ASCO   American Society of Clinical Oncology
            https://www.asco.org/news-initiatives/current-initiatives/can
            cer-care-initiatives/prevention-survivorship/survivorship-com
            pendium/care

CAPO   Canadian Association of Psychosocial Oncology,
            Recommendations for Models of Survivorship Care and
            Implementation, 2025. https://www.capo.ca/event-6141583

COSA   Clinical Oncology Society of Australia https://www.cosa.org.
            au/education-events/guidelines/

ESMO   European Society of Medical Oncology
            https://www.esmo.org/
            https://www.esmo.org/content/search?searchText=survivors
            hip+guidelines

MASCC   Multinational Association of Supportive Care in Cancer
            https://mascc.org/survivorship/

NCCN   National Comprehensive Cancer Network
            https://www.nccn.org/patients/guidelines/content/PDF/
            survivorship-hl-patient.pdf

NCI   National Cancer Institute (USA) https://cancercontrol.cancer.
            gov/ocs/special-focus-areas/national-standards-cancer-survi
            vorship-care?cid=eb_govdel

NICE   National Institute for Health and Care Excellence (UK)
            https://www.nice.org.uk/guidance/conditions-and-diseases/
            cancer

UICC   Union for International Cancer Control
            https:uicc.org

Appendix D

Resources for Training

Topic area	Source
Increase awareness and understanding of the importance of health promotion	WHO: Preventing cancer: https://www.who.int/activities/preventing-cancer
	Cancer Research UK Awareness and prevention: https://www.cancerresearchuk.org/health-professional/awareness-and-prevention
	World Cancer Research Fund: Evidence behind cancer prevention recommendations https://www.wcrf.org/research-policy/evidence-for-our-recommendations/
Identify needs and priorities that may prevent engagement in health promotion	Macmillan Cancer Support: https://www.macmillan.org.uk/healthcare-professionals/innovation-in-cancer-care/personalised-care
	NHS England PRosPER: Prehabilitation, rehabilitation, and personalized care for people living with cancer https://www.e-lfh.org.uk/programmes/prosper/
Support engagement in health promotion according to level of need	World Cancer Research Fund: Changing Behaviours: A guide on having conversations to support behavior change: https://www.wcrf.org/wp-content/uploads/2024/11/Changing-Behaviours-Guide-WEB.pdf

Index